Digested

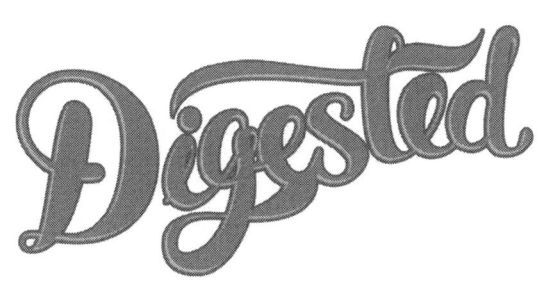

eating healthier
made easier 3 ways

• greener • allergen-free • paleo-like

Based on the experiences of an allergy-prone,
working mom who loves food (and beer)

written by Natalie Gensits

©2015 Orange Goodness LLC

All rights reserved. No part of this book may be reproduced in any form, without written permission from the copyright owner.

ISBN: 978-0-9968921-0-0

This book was intended for use as an information guide and should not be used as a substitute for professional medical care or advice. The publisher and author have made best efforts in preparing this book but make no representations or warranties with respect to the accuracy or completeness of the contents and disclaim any implied warranties of merchantability or fitness for a particular purpose. No warranty may be created or extended by sales representatives, written sales or promotional materials. The author and publisher expressly disclaim responsibility for any adverse effects arising from following advice in this book, as the advice may not be suitable for all situations. Always consult with a professional healthcare practitioner before making changes to your diet.

Dedicated to my funny, wise and loving husband, who has always encouraged me to pursue my dreams and supported me while doing so. He has weathered many diet changes for and with me — even eating gluten free for 3 weeks!

Also dedicated to my two vibrant sons, who bring joy to me every day, and my beloved pooch, Pilsner, for sharing the sunshine with me through many days of writing.

Special thanks to:

God, for calling me to embark upon this adventure and blessing me with the means to complete it.

My family — mom and stepdad, dad, brother and sister — for encouraging my efforts and playing guinea reader as needed.

Rebecca Gould, Carrie Mitchell and Laurie S. Berger, doctors of chiropractic, for the new dietary and lifestyle changes that have helped build my story. Also to Dr. Berger for showing grace and persistence through my (impatient) patient manners, and for her contributions to this book.

Dr. Mattie White, MD for reviewing and providing feedback.

Friends and contacts who have shared their "eating healthier" trials and successes in this book.

Melissa Boyster, for help with marketing strategy, insights and photography, and unwavering support both as a professional and a friend.

Steve Brumm, for designing the book cover amidst an unforgettable, amazing time in his life.

Katie Robinson, for designing and laying out the charts and book interior.

Table of contents

1. my inspiration — 1
2. establish a healthier mind-set first — 5
3. admit your motive — 7
4. understand the controversy surrounding labels and foods — 17
5. eat greener — 29
6. eat allergen free — 39
7. take a paleo-like plunge — 61
8. feed your baby more naturally — 67
9. shop smarter — 71
10. plan and prepare healthier meals — 75
11. you may not be excused — 85
12. now for dessert — sweet stories of success — 87

just one more bite — 95
your notes — 96
works cited — 99
index — 104

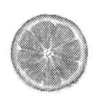

1. my inspiration

"Eating natural" and "eating healthier" have become buzz phrases. Lots of us are trying to do it. But how healthy are we really eating? Even more of us *want* to do it. But how can we eat more nutritiously with our busy lifestyles and a growing need for convenience each day? And how can we turn this trendy notion into a healthier eating nation?

These questions inspired this book. Plenty of resources — printed and online — give us recipes, theories and suggestions for eating healthier. But this book is written bearing in mind the harsh realities of how difficult eating healthier can seem, *at first*. This book is meant to simplify the concept for everyone wanting to eat healthier but especially for those who are the biggest skeptics about being able to do it. I was one of them.

I have been blessed with an amazing metabolism, so being overweight has never been an issue. During my adulthood, though, allergies — most of them environmental — have plagued me. They haven't landed me in the hospital or put me through traumatic situations. But I have high standards for how I want to feel and function, and I have lived far from those ideals. In the past 17 years, I've visited many doctors, traditional and holistic, who have been highly successful with other patients. Yet I remain a puzzle. I realize now that

I took way too many antibiotics throughout college — before learning how much harm they can do — for what I thought were sinus infections. And lately, I've struggled to recover from simple colds without a trip to the holistic doctor.

Little things have helped, but no silver bullets have surfaced, so I'm still journeying for better health and immune function. I've undergone many methods of treatment — homeopathy, enzyme treatment, acupuncture, emotional clearings, Nambudripad's Allergy Elimination Techniques (NAET) treatments, allergy shots, candida treatment and endonasal therapy, my least fave — with a slew of medical tests and cleansing diets along the way. I have learned so much about health and diet that it feels irresponsible not to share it.

The state of nutrition today is frightening and mind-blowing. Besides my own experiences trying to get healthier, other observations scream for change:

1. A growing number of traditional and holistic doctors have started to collaborate, recognizing a need for integrated treatments.

2. As a parent of two young kids, I've studied how the foods we eat can affect our health and behavioral issues — from baby cereal to ear infections, sugar to stir crazy, gluten to hyperactivity or even attention deficit hyperactivity disorder (ADHD) and autism.

3. School menus baffle me. My sons' school has taken strides in bettering menus. Still, they inevitably get 4 to 5 servings of grains before dinner. And some days they drink 2 servings of milk, 2 servings of juice and just a little water. It's shocking to see what the "norm" for kids' diets is today.

4. Cancer is rampant. Think about how many people you know who had or have cancer. More research explores the

potential link between cancer and food additives. Sites including webmd.com and sciencedaily.com mention studies that seem to verify the connection.

This book will not delve into technical or medical research about nutrition. And I am no doctor or expert. But I'm using information from my own experiences with doctors as well as other resources to make eating greener or more naturally, well, more natural. This means making it more practical and more doable, especially in a time when we are fast, furious and in need of convenience but also in demand of more energy and better health.

If just one person from a family or workplace begins to eat more naturally, seeing will encourage believing, and healthier eating can slowly become the norm again.

So, feel enlightened, dare to be entertained and prepare to encounter the word "poop" as you read, although not as frequently as I hear it, which is many times each day!

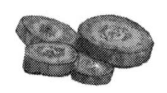

2. establish a healthier mind-set first

It's true. Research about foods, additives and illnesses is constantly changing. It will continue to change. But you have to decide if you're willing to take the risk and eat without worrying about long-term consequences. Or you may choose *not* to consume the unnatural chemicals and additives that our bodies were not designed to digest — and instead treat your body like a temple, as God intended.

When deciding to eat more naturally and prioritize your health, you should acknowledge some potential challenges to manage your expectations and "keep it real."

1. Eating naturally does not always generate *visible* positive results. I am a walking example, with a low functioning immune system and constant inflammation. And sometimes you may feel worse, *at first*. You might experience withdrawal symptoms, such as headaches, nausea, exhaustion and irritability. But hang in there, because it should level out, and this is a good indication that you need to detox. Plus, if you have several "layers" of toxicity to peel away, it will take longer to see results. After one year of eating healthier, I'm less congested — my nose isn't closing off to the point that I can barely breathe or eat at times — but I'm still struggling to feel energetic and resilient.

2. Eating naturally is not necessarily as tasty, *at first*. Sure, you can find recipes that are outstanding, but it's not as

simple as substituting stevia for sugar or buying gluten-free stuff instead of gluten-filled stuff. Rest easy knowing that your taste buds can adapt and over time, your healthier food will taste more satisfying to you.

3. Eating naturally can cost more. Health food stores make eating naturally easier, but this convenience often comes at a higher cost. However, you could save money on fewer prescriptions and doctor visits, and you could learn to feel satisfied with eating less.

4. Eating naturally takes more time and work. Think about it. When our grandparents cooked from scratch, they spent much of their day doing so. It was a full-time job. So, count on spending more time cooking.

5. Eating naturally can seem inconvenient. You may need to plan and prepare more meals ahead of time, especially if you have a full-time job.

So, why bother eating healthier?

As we grow older, we experience more aches, pains and illnesses. Our bodies aren't usually as resilient. Make a list of your current health issues and even emotional stresses. Layer on top of that the chemicals, additives and unnatural products you ingest, day after day, multiple times a day. If we take steps to remove the layers we can control, our bodies shouldn't have to work as hard to function properly.

If you need motivation, take your list and post it on the fridge. For the next week or month, every time you eat or drink something that's not so healthy, add a tick mark next to your list. Don't play dumb here. Be honest with yourself!

Next, read on for a few more reasons you might want to eat healthier.

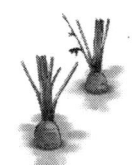

3. admit your motive

So, really, why should I go to the trouble to eat healthier, you might think?

"Because I can!" as my then 3-year old would say. While this is the best answer, there are many. As with any goal, if you can identify your motive, you will feel more encouraged and focused as you journey.

The article "Pre-diabetes, diabetes rates fuel national health crisis," published on USAtoday.com in 2014, discusses how nearly 50 percent of Americans either have diabetes or pre-diabetes, a condition marked by higher-than-normal blood sugar. Just as startling, according to the book *Why Do I Still Have Thyroid Symptoms?* by Dr. Datis Kharrazian, gastrointestinal dysfunctions are the most overlooked and common disorders today, affecting about 70 million Americans and accounting for billions of dollars in annual sales of over-the-counter digestive aids. That total doesn't even include prescription medicines.

Medications can temporarily make you feel better, but what are they doing to your body over the long term? Look at all the potential side effects listed for them. Instead of fixing digestive or other issues with unnatural substances that could secretly wreak havoc elsewhere in your body, wouldn't you rather make your body healthier? Treat it like you need it for keeps, not just temporarily.

Everyone

What goes in must come out, except for the nutrients your body absorbs when functioning properly. In a perfect world, you might poop after every meal, but you should go at least once a day. You can eat junk and take medications to move it along. Or you can eat more naturally, let your body absorb loads of nutrients to help make the rest of your organs happier, and allow the rest to filter out. Consider it a family-wide movement for healthy pooping to help prevent immune dysfunction, heart disease, diabetes, cancer, other diseases and more common problems with allergies and fatigue.

Weight-loss seekers

If you're trying to lose weight, know that many products labeled as diet or weight loss foods still contain chemicals, harmful sugar substitutes or other toxins. So, cut back on all "diet" packaged foods, and choose whole foods instead. Always get your doctor's advice when dieting to lose weight, to make sure you're getting all the nutrients your body needs to function optimally.

Older adults

You may help prevent or control arthritis and digestive issues by removing foods that can cause inflammation, such as gluten, dairy and nightshades.

Women

Eating healthy, especially eating healthy fats, helps regulate hormones, which impact your mood and prevent menopausal symptoms as well as diseases such as cancer, hypothyroidism and autoimmune disorders. Your thyroid and hormones can test normal in the labs, but that doesn't mean they're at optimal levels. And both can cause great dysfunction throughout your body.

Pregnant women or nursing moms

Your baby is demanding long before he or she is born and quickly becomes what you eat. You are eating for two, and you both benefit from eating wisely.

Men

Help ward off such conditions as arthritis, heart disease, diabetes and prostate cancer, so you can keep up with your kids and set a good example. If your wife or kids need to avoid certain foods, your support makes it so much easier for them.

30-somethings

This may be your last chance to increase your bone density, according to Geoff Bond in his book *Natural Eating, Nutritional Anthropology*. You can do this by adding vitamins K and D to your diet, along with calcium and potassium, while reducing your intake of alcohol and caffeine. You've had plenty of time to be young and, well, less responsible! Now is the time to set yourself up for better health, as you approach mid-life hormonal changes. It's a great time to set good examples for the kids in your life, too.

Kids

Today, 1 of 3 kids is at risk to develop adult-onset diabetes, also called type 2 diabetes, according to Sarah Fragoso in *Everyday Paleo*. More kids are becoming obese. More kids are being diagnosed with attention deficit disorder (ADD) or hyperactivity and being medicated for it. Over the long-term, these medications can cause or worsen chronic allergies, sinus problems or digestive issues.

Yet kids are so impressionable, so why not instill natural eating habits in them now, before they get set in unhealthy ways? Sure, they may stray from good eating habits in later, rebellious years. But chances are they will come back to them eventually and thank you for the healthier foundation you established during their upbringings. Plus, you're providing damage control during a crucial time of growth and development for them.

So, how does food and digestion relate to your overall health anyhow?

In a nutshell, our bodies digest the food we eat to provide energy and the other nutrients we need to function properly. Our organs, bones, muscles and nerves rely on digestion to help prevent deficiencies, sicknesses and conditions that often lead to disease.

Digestion gets complex, but I've referenced articles on enchantedlearning.com and livescience.com and will simplify it even further here.

1. Digestion begins in your mouth as you chew, with the help of your salivary enzymes.

2. Your esophagus carries food from your mouth to your stomach.

3. Your stomach immerses the food in gastric (stomach) acid and starts breaking down protein while killing harmful bacteria.

4. In the small intestine, bile, pancreatic enzymes and other digestive enzymes further break down your food. Most nutrient absorption occurs in your small intestine, and those are then moved into your bloodstream and taken to your liver.

5. Your liver converts nutrients to energy and breaks down unwanted chemicals, such as alcohol, so they can be excreted or extracted from your body.

6. Remaining materials travel to your large intestine (colon), where water and electrolytes are removed. Storage of indigestible materials also occurs here.

7. These indigestible materials are excreted when you poop or may become toxic inside your body when you don't poop often enough.

To sum it up, when your body isn't digesting properly, it may not be getting the nutrition it needs and it may not be getting rid of the waste it doesn't need.

Digestive details not talked about often enough

By digging just a little more into the details of our digestive systems, we can better visualize and appreciate how it works and its significance in our overall health.

1. Your nutrient-absorbing small intestine contains digestive flora, which can become unbalanced due to use of antibiotics, birth control pills, hormones (including steroids) and alcohol. Stress and diet can also disrupt the balance.

2. Mucous membranes are key to protecting you from harmful microbes and parasites that can cause infection. They are found throughout your body — in your nose, mouth, lungs and urinary digestive tract. Many infections and diseases can begin as, or can be related to, inflammation in your mucous membranes — allergies, asthma and sinusitis, angioedema, arthritis, bronchitis, influenza, lymphoma and the list goes on. By eating to prevent or reduce inflammation in your body, you help your mucous membranes do their job.

3. Intestinal villi are projections in your digestive mucous membranes that allow the absorption of nutrients. For example, when a person with celiac disease, a digestive intolerance to gluten, eats gluten, her body will react allergically, possibly for several days. Her body may also damage the villi, hindering their ability to absorb nutrients properly.

So, eating even a little bit of a "culprit food," one that causes a visible or invisible bodily reaction, can seem to cause only an annoying but tolerable reaction, like minor itching or stuffiness. In reality, each time you eat it, you can damage your body's digestive system. Damage to your intestinal flora, mucous membranes or villi can serve as a root to other problems. And the more damage that's done, the harder it can be and longer it can take to repair it.

So, maybe now, you are encouraged. Or overwhelmed. Or both. I'm not one to sugarcoat because confronting reality helps me digest it into more manageable parts. Eating naturally can take a lot of time and work. It can even cause stress and exhaustion for you, like it did me, at first. But now, even though I don't eat paleo or perfectly otherwise, I've adapted a lot of habits to eat more naturally. Now I do them without thinking twice and without missing my old ways.

- *I rarely eat gluten for breakfast or dinner. For breakfast, I eat some variation of eggs, homemade sausage and/or sweet potatoes.*
- *For lunch, I often eat leftovers, a salad or sometimes a sandwich on gluten-free, organic bread.*
- *For snacks, I stick to fresh fruits or vegetables, olives, sometimes cheese, sweet potato chips or other healthier (not necessarily healthy) versions of gluten-free chips.*

> - *For dinner, I usually forgo bread, even with a hamburger.*
> - *I still eat out occasionally.*
> - *In general, I limit my intake of grains, starches or carbs and dairy. I still enjoy some gluten, but usually in the form of a beer and just one or two at a sitting.*
>
> I should add that the reason I don't eat totally gluten free or paleo is that I've done spurts of each and didn't get the results that others have experienced. I'm still working on improving my energy and allergies through healthier eating, though, because it takes some people longer to heal than others, and I have several layers to peel away.
>
> I admit that I've worked as a freelance writer while making these changes to my eating habits, so my schedule has been more flexible. But I've had two young kids in school and daycare while I've worked full-time or part-time. My husband works full-time. I love food and a good beer as much as anyone. And I have a man-like appetite to keep up with, which is not easy when you limit the filling grains and starches! So, if I can make changes to eat healthier, you can, too.

And there's a good chance you'll feel better for it. Most people I know who've eaten healthier and even gluten free have experienced positive results, usually in just a couple of weeks.

Strategize to make it easier on yourself. If you have any hesitations, do it during a time when you have less stress and activity, so this doesn't add to your frustration. For example, avoid making changes during a move, a vacation or your period. Take the plunge or start with baby steps if it helps you feel less overwhelmed.

Remember that accountability comes with commitment. You need to remind yourself during this transition that you have chosen this path for your specific reasons. Seriously, write your reasons down and hang them up. Your list will help to combat moments of frustration.

When you've come to terms with the challenges and decide that you are ready to eat even a little more naturally, this book will help puree big steps into digestible bits. This book is crafted to help you eat healthier no matter which level you're at:

- **Eat greener, chapter 5:** You're not looking for major overhauls but would like to make some wiser choices without revamping your lifestyle.
- **Eat allergen free, chapter 6:** You want to use diet instead of drugs to help heal your body and/or you wish to avoid compounding food sensitivities.
- **Take a paleo-like plunge, chapter 7:** You want to eat extremely organically or caveman-style with chemical-free meats, fruits and vegetables and without grains or dairy.

> *I fall somewhere in the allergen-free category. I've experienced and seen my kids experience troubles from eating too many grains or too much dairy. I've grown sensitive to some foods as well as additives like yellow 5 in the past few years. And I've eaten paleo-like as a cleansing effort but without major results.*
>
> *Meanwhile, I have two young kids who I hope grow up to be healthy and without chronic allergies. I don't want to spend my career in the kitchen and at grocery stores, but I do spend ample time and money to eat and feed my family more naturally. Since we don't have full-blown food allergies, we don't have to avoid anything completely. Instead, I aim to eat foods that irritate in moderation, if at all.*

> *For a frame of reference or perspective, I believe:*
> - *Genetically modified organisms (GMOs) are likely a contributing cause of cancer and shortened lives.*
> - *Grains are often a source of GMOs, often difficult to digest and unnecessary.*
> - *Excess amounts of gluten can constipate, agitate and cause hyperactivity, lack of focus or irritability.*
> - *Soy is difficult for some to digest, so I generally avoid it.*
> - *Raw sugar is better than sweeteners and unnatural substitutes.*
> - *Lean meats are good, in moderation.*
> - *You should drink mostly water, every day. Aim to drink at least half your weight in ounces daily, and more when exercising or during extreme heat.*
> - *Plastic containers could be contributing to diseases and illnesses.*

Note that my beliefs are just that — beliefs based on my own body, experiences and research. I'm not saying they are right or perfect. I will not try to convince you to believe the same. But I am sharing them to give you a clearer picture of my reality and to demonstrate that regardless of your beliefs, you can find ways to eat more naturally that work for you.

Be hopeful. Eating healthier seems more difficult in the beginning, but it should get much easier over time. Life is not all about food, even though it kinda is. Eating should be more of a survival act than one for entertainment, meaning you eat the essentials and not just whatever's convenient or tasty. And by eating more naturally, you can hope to attain better health and greater happiness in life.

Enjoy, and may you easily digest!

4. understand the controversy surrounding labels and foods

Breaking down confusion about labels

Food labels have become more confusing, and many terms have become buzzwords. Take "whole grain" as an example. Many brands, schools and restaurants promote their use of "whole grains" as a health benefit. Though the product may contain some whole grains, it may also contain genetically modified organisms, also known as GMOs, which diminish the value of the whole grains and the overall product.

This section will be helpful while shopping and will add meaning to the next few chapters. So, let's sort through some basics about food labels. Defining some of these terms is like hitting a moving target, or brushing a 2-year-old's teeth, because products and research seem to change constantly. Be aware that these definitions, as they relate to food labels, may change over time. But those changes would be welcome if they resulted in food labels becoming more heavily monitored.

First, **genetic modification** is the process of forcing genes from one species into another unrelated species and is also known as genetic engineering (gmo-awareness.com 2011-2014). We find many foods with GMOs, which are thought to contribute to the outlandish amount of cancer and disease we see today. According to gmo-awareness.com, the Big Four GMO crops are corn, soy, canola oil and cottonseed oil.

Whole foods are considered healthy, according to merriam-webster.com, because they're grown naturally, have not been processed and contain no artificial ingredients.

The term **organic** gets a little more complicated, so I'm providing definitions directly from the United States Department of Agriculture's website. Note that the following terms are listed from most to least organic.

For food products to be **certified organic by the United States Department of Agriculture (USDA)**, they must be:

- produced without excluded methods, such as genetic engineering, ionizing radiation or sewage sludge.

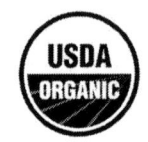

- produced per the National List of Allowed and Prohibited Substances.

- overseen by a USDA National Organic Program-authorized certifying agent, following all USDA organic regulations.

For **organic crops**, the USDA organic seal verifies that irradiation, sewage sludge, synthetic fertilizers, prohibited pesticides and genetically modified organisms were not used.

For **organic livestock,** the USDA organic seal verifies that producers met animal health and welfare standards, did not use antibiotics or growth hormones, used 100% organic feed and provided animals with access to the outdoors.

Raw or processed agricultural products in the **100 percent certified organic** category must meet these criteria:

- ✓ All ingredients must be certified organic.
- ✓ Any processing aids must be organic.
- ✓ Product labels must state the name of the certifying agent on the information panel.

- ✓ The principal display panel may include the USDA organic seal and/or 100 percent organic claim.
- ✓ The information panel must identify organic ingredients (e.g., organic dill) or via asterisk or other mark.

For **organic multi-ingredient foods**, such as packaged goods, the USDA organic seal verifies that the product has 95% or more certified organic content. If the label claims that it was made with specified organic ingredients, you can be sure that those specific ingredients are certified organic.

Organic raw or processed agricultural products must meet these criteria, set by the USDA:

- ✓ All agricultural ingredients must be certified organic, except where specified on the National List.
- ✓ Non-organic ingredients allowed per the National List may be used, up to a combined total of five percent of non-organic content, excluding salt and water.
- ✓ Product labels must state the name of the certifying agent on the information panel.
- ✓ The principal display panel may include the USDA organic seal and/or organic claim.
- ✓ The information panel must identify organic ingredients (e.g., organic dill) or via asterisk or other mark.

While the **Non-GMO Project verified** seal is not a GMO-free claim, it assures that the product has been produced according to *consensus-based best practices* for GMO avoidance. The Project's website, nongmoproject.org, claims that the group is North America's only independent verification for products made according to best practices for GMO avoidance.

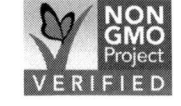

The bottom line? Products with "organic" written on, or incorporated into, the packaging may not have been subjected to regulatory testing. Some foods with "organic" on the labels may contain both organic and non-organic ingredients. By looking for the "USDA organic" and "Non-GMO Project verified" seals, you can hope that you are getting more organic products.

As stated by USDA, meat, poultry and egg products labeled as **"natural"** must be minimally processed and contain no artificial ingredients. However, the natural label does not include any standards regarding farm practices and applies only to processing of meat and egg products. There are no standards or regulations for the labeling of natural food products if they do not contain meat or eggs.

For other foods, the Food and Drug Administration (FDA) stated in 2015: "it is difficult to define a food product that is 'natural' because the food has probably been processed and is no longer the product of the earth. That said, FDA has not developed a definition for use of the term natural or its derivatives. However, the agency has not objected to the use of the term if the food does not contain added color, artificial flavors, or synthetic substances."

Because the term seems rather loosely regulated and defined, I give little if any weight to products with "natural" on the labels. If you consider buying them, closely inspect the ingredients list first.

The following labels describe how animals were raised and were taken directly from USDA's Agricultural Marketing Service website. Note, though, that these standards do not address whether the animals were fed hormones or antibiotics.

For **grass-fed** animals, grass and forage shall be the feed source consumed for the lifetime of the ruminant animal, with the exception of milk consumed prior to weaning. The diet shall be derived solely from forage consisting of grass (annual and perennial), forbs (e.g., legumes, Brassica), browse or cereal grain crops in the vegetative (pre-grain) state. Animals cannot be fed grain or grain byproducts and must have continuous access to pasture during the growing season. Hay, haylage, baleage, silage, crop residue without grain and other roughage sources may also be included as acceptable feed sources. Routine mineral and vitamin supplementation may also be included in the feeding regimen. If incidental supplementation occurs due to inadvertent exposure to non-forage feedstuffs or to ensure the animal's well being at all times during adverse environmental or physical conditions, the producer must fully document (e.g., receipts, ingredients and tear tags) the supplementation that occurs including the amount, the frequency and the supplements provided.

Pasture-raised animals must have had continuous, free access to the out-of-doors for a significant portion of their lives.

Free-range animals were provided shelter in a building, room or area with unlimited access to food, fresh water and continuous access to the outdoors during their production cycle. The outdoor area may or may not have been fenced and/or covered with netting-like material.

Cage-free animals were able to freely roam a building, room or enclosed area with unlimited access to food and fresh water during their production cycle.

Be aware that conventional meat and poultry animals are often fed GMO grains that were grown using pesticides or other chemicals. So, for meat or poultry, it's best to look for "USDA organic," "hormone and antibiotic-free" and "grass-fed" on the labels if you want the purest form without grains.

Labels on grain products can be confusing, too.

Multi-grain means that more than one grain is used and does not indicate that it's whole grain or organic.

Whole grain indicates that all parts of the grain kernel — bran, germ and endosperm — are used, as defined by the Whole Grains Council in "Identifying Whole Grain Products." The bran and germ are the key providers of nutrients. In contrast, white bread is made using only the endosperm, which explains why whole grains are more nutritious. However, many products labeled "whole grain" contain other grains that aren't whole, too.

100% whole grain means all parts of the grain kernel — bran, germ and endosperm — are used for all of the grains in that product, according to the Whole Grains Council.

The Whole Grains Council "100%" stamp means the product contains only grains that are whole, but it may contain many other ingredients and does not mean the product is organic.

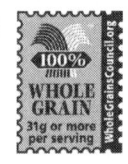

Labels can deceive. The term "natural" lacks regulation. Even products with "organic" scripted on the label often contain non-organic ingredients, too. Other labels make claims that entice, such as "with juice concentrate," when that could just be a way of adding sugar unnecessarily.

Reading labels requires diligence, caution and a certain amount of trust in the regulating standards and processes. So, shopping organic and eating healthier can take more time in the beginning, but they get easier with practice and understanding.

Understanding the controversy about certain foods

One year, eggs are a health risk. The next, they are good for you again. We hear about foods in the news more often, as research is being done constantly. And we can find tons of information online, although distinguishing what's right or true isn't easy. This section sums up recent or current controversy surrounding several foods.

Grains are ... a little grainy

You'll find much controversy about grains and gluten, suggesting connections to cancer, ADD, ADHD, thyroid issues and more. But one thing is certain. Breads are not what they used to be — not during biblical times and not in our grandparents' times, as noted in Geoff Bond's *Natural Eating, Nutritional Anthropology*. Bond discusses how bread used to be made without GMOs and with only 100% whole grains, yeast and maybe a pinch of salt.

Now, GMOs are often added to bread to mass-produce it more quickly while making it lighter and less chewy. But these GMOs can cause health issues. The growing number of people with gluten intolerances causes us to wonder if the intolerance has developed due to the gluten or all the GMOs! We will cover more about this in the *Eat allergen free* chapter.

So, be aware that many packaged breads contain gluten and GMOs. While shopping, avoid products with enriched, bleached or unbleached flour and instead look for labels such as:

- 100% organic whole grain.
- 100% organic sprouted or seed made without flours.
- "Non-GMO Project Verified."

Also note that because many of these breads do not contain additives, they often require refrigeration after opening, if not all the time.

Both traditional and holistic doctors will likely encourage you to choose 100% whole grains that are not "enriched" or "bleached" in moderation — organic is even better. Holistic doctors may even favor avoidance of them. If you're interested in reducing grains in your diet, you will find substitutes and other sources of fiber in the *Eat allergen free* chapter.

> *I eat grains in moderation and have decided to buy 100% organic bread or gluten-free seed bread whenever possible, since it is a staple for lunches and our main source of grain. Meanwhile, we've greatly reduced other sources of grains, such as pizza and pasta, to 3 – 4 times per month combined. When we eat pasta, we choose noodles made from brown rice, black bean or quinoa instead of 100% whole wheat to avoid another dose of gluten.*

The dairy low-down

Dairy tends to be more difficult to digest, both literally and figuratively, and you'll find great debate over it. First, if you're sensitive to casein, a milk protein, you are likely to have difficulty digesting any type of animal milk.

In fact, sensitivity to casein can trigger autoimmune responses, just as gluten can. This means your enzymes are not properly digesting the protein, and your body goes into attack mode as if it's fighting a virus. Over time, this autoimmune response can cause more serious problems or diseases. So, if you've been diagnosed with an autoimmune disease, you may want to avoid dairy.

Casein issue aside, if your body does not have sufficient lactase, the enzyme that breaks down lactose, you could be lactose intolerant. Some online sources say people who have been deemed lactose intolerant, as opposed to outright *allergic* to dairy, can possibly drink milk from sheep or goats because it contains smaller fat globules, and more medium-chain fatty acids, making it easier to digest.

Other lactose-intolerant people can consume *raw* milk more easily, because it has not been pasteurized or homogenized. Pasteurized milk has been heated to a high temperature to kill potentially disease-producing microorganisms, but this process also kills the enzymes that help you digest it while damaging its vitamin and mineral content. That's why some health experts believe raw milk provides more nutrients. However, the Centers for Disease Control and Prevention (CDC) warns that you risk getting sick from raw milk because it's not pasteurized.

Homogenization breaks down the fat globules in milk so that they do not separate as cream, but the fat particles can become so small that they enter your blood stream without being digested. This can contribute to milk allergies or intolerances.

Regarding how the animals were fed, you can choose milk from animals that have been fed only grasses, as some research suggests that it contains higher levels of fat-soluble vitamins, nutrients and conjugated linoleic acid (CLA). CLA might help reduce body fat deposits and improve immune function, according to webmd.com.

If you drink milk from grain-fed animals, you could expose yourself to chemicals, such as pesticides and herbicides that are used to grow the grain, in addition to the grains themselves — not good if you're trying to avoid or limit grain intake.

You also can opt for organic dairy products. But organic milk may be pasteurized and/or homogenized.

In the end, your milk and dairy choices will depend on your priorities, beliefs and responses. Do your own research and consult with your doctor to decide what's best for you and your family.

> My family seldom drinks milk at home. We occasionally use it for cereal or recipes, so I usually buy organic milk. We eat some cheeses and organic or Greek yogurt without additives or sugar substitutes. Eventually, I'd like to get even healthier with our dairy choices, but for now, I'm focusing on the foods we eat in mass quantities.

Soy drama

Soy is also under the scope. Considered by health experts as a good source of protein, soy provides fiber, vitamin K, iron, magnesium, phosphorus and copper. It can help regulate cholesterol and cell growth. But soy is difficult for some to digest and an allergen for others. Some research links soy to hormone imbalance issues, possibly speeding up the maturation of kids and contributing to infertility issues for women.

If you can easily digest soy, choose 100% organic soy, tofu or immature beans known as edamame without added sugars, evaporated cane juice or brown rice syrup. Or choose 100% organic, fermented products like miso, natto or tempeh, which also provide your body with natural probiotics.

Avoid soy milk with far-out expiration dates, since it will likely contain additives. Also avoid soy or soy protein in bars or other pre-packaged foods, such as some fake meat or dairy products, as they are often processed and stripped of nutrients.

Then keep soy on your radar as more research gets published about it — as any risk may have more to do with the quality and quantity consumed rather than the food itself.

> My family doesn't eat soy except for some occasional edamame, as I don't seem to digest it well. We get plenty of protein from eggs, lean meats and beans.

Sugar and high fructose corn syrup situation

Controversy continues to circulate over the effects of high fructose corn syrup (HFCS). It's considered unnatural because producing it involves adding enzymes and altering regular corn syrup's molecular content, meaning it's genetically modified. Some sources think HFCS contributes to fat deposits in your liver, which can lead to plaque build-up and narrowed blood vessels. Research also indicates that regular sugar calms hunger hormones while HFCS makes you feel unable to satisfy your hunger, which could encourage overeating.

Food companies use HFCS because it's cheaper to produce and we have a large supply of corn. You'll find high fructose corn syrup in sodas, fruit juices and other sweetened drinks, baked goods, canned fruits and dairy items.

Despite the controversy, one thing is certain. Too much added sugar, whatever the source, adds calories to your diet, which can contribute to weight gain and health problems including type 2 diabetes and metabolic syndrome. Each increases your risk for heart disease.

> *I usually avoid fruit drinks, canned fruit or other products with high or low fructose corn syrup. Instead, I'll buy canned pears in 100% juice and pure maple syrup. Occasionally, I have a soda or let the kids eat Halloween candy containing corn syrup. My theory is that striving for perfection tends to add stress and tempt greater rebellion, especially from kids. If I allow my kids to eat unnatural or unhealthy foods sparingly and explain why, they will hopefully maintain better eating habits as they grow more independent, without feeling resentful or deprived now.*

Prioritizing these food dilemmas takes some personal exploration or trial and error, as our bodies all work in unique ways. So, let's talk about some basic changes you can make to eat healthier, regardless of how those priorities stack up for you.

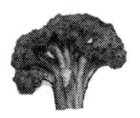

5. eat greener

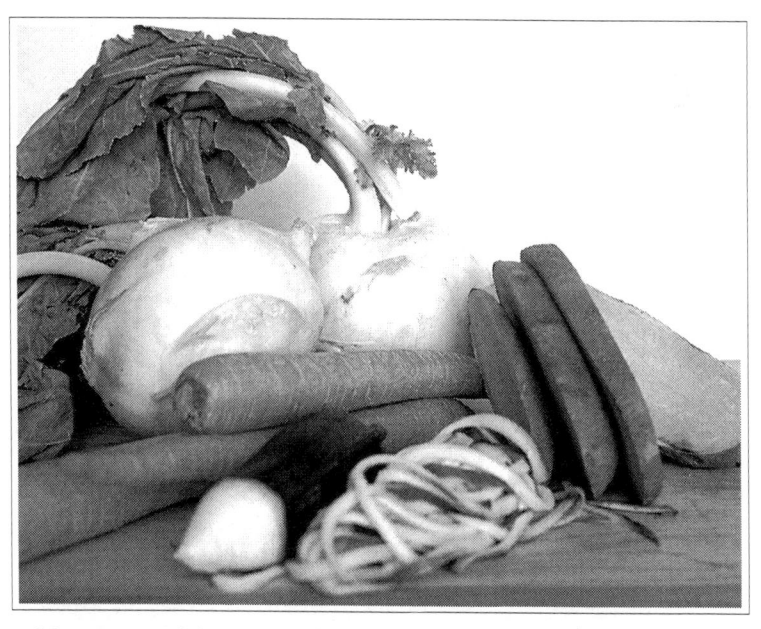

Add variety with less common vegetables like kohlrabi. Serve carrots, zucchini and sweet potatoes in non-typical fashion.

If you admit that you're far from ready to make a serious paleo-like change to your diet and lifestyle but want to take a few steps to eat more naturally, you'll find plenty of options in this chapter. Following are some basic changes you can make to your diet to eat healthier.

① Add lots of vegetables to your diet. Aim to make 50% of the foods you eat vegetables that are rich in nutrients and organically grown.

- Replace starchy potatoes with sweet potatoes, even for breakfast. Sauté, bake, mash or grill sweet potatoes for different textures because *white* potatoes are a member of a group of foods called nightshades (p. 48). These foods contain alkaloids, which can promote inflammation while hindering joint movement or digestion.

- Limit other starchy, poop-stopping options such as peas, most beans (except green) and corn, which is actually a grain. Instead, choose easier to digest veggies including carrots, squash, zucchini and Swiss chard. Try peppers and eggplant, if you tolerate nightshades.

- Replace low-nutrient iceberg lettuce with darker green and red leaf lettuce. The more color, the more nutrients.

② Eat organic foods. Remember that "100% organic" is better than "organic." Organic foods are more expensive than non-organic, but you often can find better prices at farmers' markets. Or, consider growing your own and start a garden swap with your neighbors. Choose organic:

- fruits and vegetables to help avoid exposure to pesticides or other harmful chemicals. If you have to prioritize what produce you buy organic, put foods with edible flesh first — bell peppers, tomatoes, leafy greens, peaches, cherries, pears, strawberries, blueberries and apples. They are thin-skinned and typically sprayed more often than other fruits and vegetables. Produce without edible flesh, such as squash, bananas and oranges, could be less exposed to chemicals.

- grains to avoid GMOs. When prioritizing in this food group, opt for organic versions of staple grain items such as bread or pasta. Also select 100% organic versions of any products containing the Big Four crops — corn, soy, canola oil and cottonseed oil.

- proteins, including lean meats, sausages and deli meats, with minimal nitrates or nitrites, in which the animals were grass-fed, pasture-raised or free-range. Meat from wild animals tends to be better for you than meat from animals raised on a farm because farm animals could have been fed GMO-containing grains that were treated with chemicals or pesticides. So, if you find organic, grass-fed, pasture-raised or free-range product labels that also say the animals were *not* grain-fed, even better!

③ Opt for organic, free-range eggs and dairy products, such as organic milk or certified organic ghee clarified butter, in which the animals were not fed hormones, GMO-containing grains or medicines.

④ Limit soy products. Although soy has become a major player in allergy-based or vegetarian-based diets, not everyone can digest it easily and not all soy products are healthy. Many contain GMOs or hormones, so choose only 100% organic soy products or edamame, which are baby beans.

⑤ Add probiotics. Our bodies naturally produce probiotics, but many factors can affect them, including:

- consuming food additives, food colorings and sugars.
- consuming processed foods.
- drinking water with chlorine and/or fluoride.
- taking antibiotics.
- using antiseptic sprays and soaps.
- inhaling air pollution.

Probiotics help keep your intestinal flora balanced. When not balanced, any resulting inflammation can lead to many conditions, including depression, irritable bowel syndrome, autoimmune disorders or leaky gut syndrome (p. 44), just to name a few.

Both traditional and holistic doctors are turning more frequently to supplemental probiotics, in capsules or powders, to maintain the good bacteria in the digestive system. Especially if you have digestive issues, such as IBS or constipation, a daily dose of probiotics can make a noticeable difference in your bowel movements and how you feel.

Probiotics are a no-brainer if you feel run down, are travelling or must resort to taking antibiotics. Sources vary, but some say it can take your digestive system a year to recover from just one round of antibiotics. At times, antibiotics are necessary, but they can also kill the good bacteria you need for a healthy, balanced immune system.

You can also get probiotics from unsweetened, organic goat, sheep or coconut yogurt without sugar or sugar substitutes or from fermented foods, such as kimchi and some sauerkraut. You can usually find these in the refrigerated section of health food stores. Choose products that do not contain vinegar, which can hinder natural fermentation. Make sure they do not contain other additives and that they have not been pasteurized, which can kill the beneficial probiotic bacteria.

⑥ Drink more water. Water prevents and helps heal inflammation while supporting your immune system, cardiovascular health, skin and digestive system. Be aware, though, that drinking ridiculously excessive amounts of water, after playing endurance sports, for example, can dilute your electrolytes and cause serious complications like hyponatremia, which can lead to confusion, seizures, coma and death. You can ask your doctor for a recommendation based on your personal lifestyle and habits, but a good rule of thumb is to divide your weight in half and drink at least that many ounces of water daily. If it's extremely hot, you work out or you consume lots of caffeine, drink more water, as these tend to dehydrate you.

- Keep a refillable glass bottle in your car, one at work and a glass at home. Filtered or purified water rules, because the chlorine in tap water can kill off the good bacteria in your body, which will counter your efforts to add probiotics.

- Avoid drinking water — or eating food — that has been heated by the sun or microwave in plastic containers made with bisphenol A (BPA). Some studies suggest that BPA can be released into foods or water when heated, possibly producing estrogen-like effects, which may also increase your risk for cancer. Newer studies indicate that *freezing* water in BPA-containing plastic could cause similar effects.

- If you get bored with plain water, flavor it with a squeeze of fresh lime or lemon. Or add a splash of organic, unsweetened fruit juice.

> *I have 2 cups of herbal black tea in the morning and otherwise drink water, with an occasional beer or glass of red wine in the evenings or on weekends. My kids drink primarily water at home, with occasional milk or junk-free fruit juice. They get a serving of milk and/or fruit juice at school, but they take a full reusable bottle of filtered water with them each day.*

(7) Remove the salt shaker from your table. Yes, sodium helps to regulate your body's water balance, while controlling your muscle and nerve function and supporting your circulatory system. And if you are active or sweat a lot, you may want to consume slightly more than the recommended daily amount of sodium. But according to fda.gov, Americans eat on average about 3,300 milligrams of salt per day. The Dietary Guidelines for Americans recommend consuming less than 2,300 milligrams per day, which is equal to about 1 teaspoon. African-Americans, people over age 51 or people with conditions including high blood pressure, diabetes or chronic kidney disease should consume no more than 1,500 milligrams of sodium per day. Too much sodium can also worsen congestive heart failure.

Many of us could benefit from reducing our daily sodium consumption. If you need to reduce your sodium intake, choose whole foods instead of packaged foods and remove the salt shaker from your table so you'll be less tempted to use it.

When you add salt, opt for Himalayan crystal salt in moderation. Many health experts consider it the healthiest salt because it was mined before oceans became so polluted and provides minerals, trace elements and other health benefits. Otherwise, you can get sodium naturally from salt-water fish, meat, sea vegetables, beets, carrots, celery and spinach.

(8) Sever your attachment to sweets. Sugar does not provide nutrients for your body. Although whole veggies and fruits contain natural sugars such as fructose or sugar cane, other foods contain refined, or processed sugars, including high fructose and low fructose corn syrup (p. 27), malto-dextrin, dextrose, sucrose, maltose, glucose, evaporated cane juice, caramel, fruit juice and carob syrup. Or they may contain sugar substitutes, such as Splenda, galactose, aspartame or sorbitol, which are found in many sodas and yogurts and thought to potentially cause cancer, although research is not conclusive at this point.

Besides cancer, which is scary enough, many processed sugars seem to be linked to a slew of other health issues, including acne, allergies, behavioral problems, bloating, cancer, cardiovascular disease, constipation, depression, fatigue, food cravings, high cholesterol and triglycerides, hypoglycemia, immune dysfunction, indigestion, mental illness, muscle pain, obesity, premenstrual syndrome (PMS), type 2 diabetes, ulcers and yeast infection.

The bottom line is that artificial sweeteners may cause more harm than good, as discussed in Dr. Joseph Mercola's article "Sugar Substitutes — What's Safe and What's Not."

The American Heart Association recommends that women get no more than 100 calories per day from added sugar from any source and that most men get no more than 150 calories per day from added sugar. This equates to about 6 teaspoons for women and 9 teaspoons for men.

However, the average U.S. adult consumes 22 teaspoons of sugar daily, and the average child takes in 32 teaspoons per day. If you want more jaw-dropping details about sugar consumption, check out "How Much Sugar Are Americans Eating?" by Alice Walton on Forbes.com.

As a frame of reference, use these few examples of common foods and how much sugar they contain from "How much sugar is in your food?" by Joseph Nordqvist on medicalnewstoday.com.

Examples of sugar content

pack of M&Ms	5.75 tsp
Snickers	7.0 tsp
100 grams of marshmallows	14.5 tsp
fruit smoothie	3.5 tsp
12-oz. can Coca-Cola	7.0 tsp
Red Bull	7.5 tsp
Cheerios	1.1 tsp
Honey Nut Cheerios	8.25 tsp
Cocoa Puffs	9.3 tsp
Fruit Loops	10.6 tsp
100 grams of blueberries	1.7 tsp
100 grams of banana	3.0 tsp
100 grams of grapes	4.0 tsp
1 scoop ice cream	3.0 tsp
1 jam doughnut	3.5 tsp
1 chocolate chip muffin	4.75 tsp

Note that 100 grams is equivalent to just less than ½ cup, or .42268 c, to be exact.

When you do consume sugar, consider:

- using raw or organic sugar, or organic sweeteners such as stevia, honey, xylitol or brown rice syrup, in moderation.
- buying organic maple syrup instead of syrups with high fructose corn syrup.
- buying canned fruits in fruit juices or water instead of syrup.
- avoiding synthetic sugar substitutes, such as Splenda, galactose, glucose, aspartame and sorbitol, which are found in many yogurts and sodas.

- giving up the soda or saving it for an occasional treat.

- removing sugary treats as rewards for your kids. Give them something natural and sweet, like fresh fruit if it must be food. Or reward them with an extra book, extra playtime or a family silly dance session instead. Be creative and try to leave food out of the bribe equation!

9. Opt for organic coffee because non-organic coffee is typically sprayed with fertilizers, pesticides or other chemicals. If the coffee is grown outside the U.S., however, proving that it's been grown using organic standards is difficult. If you choose decaffeinated coffee, look for brands that use the chemical-free Swiss Water process, because even products with "naturally decaffeinated" on the label may be exposed to chemicals in the process.

For drip coffee makers, use unbleached filters to avoid chlorine, which can destroy your good intestinal bacteria, those natural probiotics.

10. Overhaul your snacks. Since we're so mobile these days, overhaul your snack cupboard or drawer to include healthier yet still convenient options.

- Throw out the candy and cookies, or keep one choice that's organic without all the additives.

- Keep a stash of fresh cut carrot sticks, celery sticks, peppers or cucumbers, as well as berries, grapes, bananas and apples to replace crackers and potato chips. Cut and wash veggies as soon as you buy them, so you'll be more likely to eat them.

- Stock up with organic applesauce packets, many of which include kale or other vegetables. I'm not sure these are a perfect solution. The long shelf life concerns me, but I'm hopeful these are healthier than chips, cookies and crackers!

- If you insist on serving snack bars, buy versions with organic ingredients or at least without additives.

- Avoid fruit snacks or other foods with dyes (yellow 5, blue 3, red 5, etc.). Yellow 5, also called tartrazine, can cause allergic responses or intolerances in some people and hyperactivity in some kids.

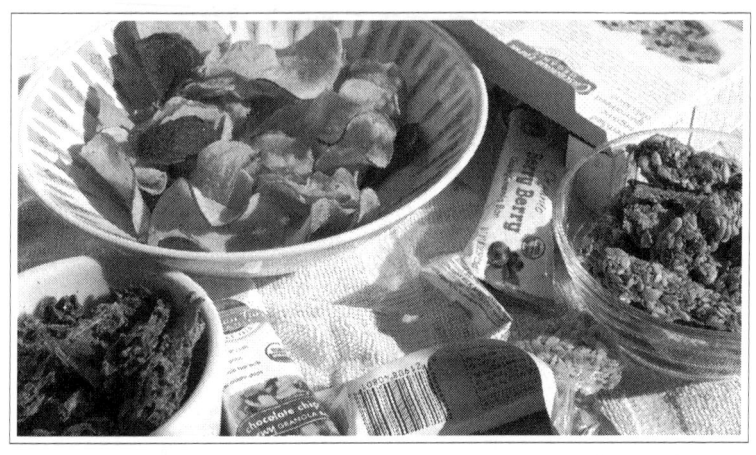

Fill your snack drawer with organic kale or sweet potato chips and nuts and seeds snacks that are healthier than crackers, chips and cookies.

We have just covered 10 ways to eat greener with specific suggestions for each. By choosing some of these steps, maybe starting with one and adding another each week, you can get your family on a healthier eating plan without feeling overwhelmed.

Now, if you dare to go one step further, or need help eating healthy while avoiding food allergens, grab a healthy snack and keep reading.

6. eat allergen free

If you have food allergies, avoidance is your easiest fix. But if the food is one you truly love, it's not that easy. And many times, your body can't tolerate healthy foods, which can really be frustrating!

Or maybe you suffer from environmental or seasonal allergies to mold, dust mites or pollen that you're trying to minimize.

If you choose to eat healthier, you could give your body a big enough break from an overload of allergens, allow your digestive system to heal and, with a doctor's advice and supervision, eventually reintroduce some of the foods without any problem. Plus, you might eliminate or at least alleviate your non-food allergies.

First, let's try to simplify allergies and food issues.

- You could have food allergies.
- You could have food intolerances or toxicities.
- Other environmental or seasonal allergies could make you prone to developing food sensitivities, be it an allergy, intolerance or toxicity.
- Food allergies can intensify your other allergies and vice versa.

With a **food allergy**, your immune system sees the food as an enemy and launches an attack on it with an antibody called

Immunoglobulin E (IgE). A food allergy can create a minor, major or even life-threatening response to just inhaling a food or eating a small piece of it. The life-threatening response, also known as anaphylaxis, can include difficult breathing, dizziness or loss of consciousness.

A **food intolerance**, however, occurs in your digestive system when you can't properly digest the food. It can cause a range of bodily responses from minor discomfort to misery. Food intolerances can stem from sensitivities to additives and chemicals or from a lack of enzymes in your system.

Food allergy or intolerance symptoms can include cough, dark circles under your eyes, flu-like fatigue, headache, hives, irregular bowel movements, irritability, itchy or prickly throat, joint pain, muscle soreness, rash, sinus issues or stomach pains. So, you may blame other "bugs" or circumstances such as poor sleep for your symptoms when, in fact, you are having a reaction to the foods you eat. In some cases, the more cravings you have for a particular food, the more likely it is to be an irritant.

Identifying your culprit foods — the foods that cause problems — is key, so you can avoid them or at least eat them in moderation in the case of food sensitivity, as opposed to an outright allergy. You may be able to reintroduce them after your body heals from fighting off the army of enemies it's been exposed to for so long.

If you get allergy testing, your doctor will likely test the IgE response, which is the most obvious and severe response. However, to get a true reading of your food *intolerances*, too, find a doctor that will perform an IgG allergy test, which can detect foods that may be secretly beating you up over time with delayed or subtle symptoms.

In holistic health, your doctor may detect a **food toxicity**. Think of a toxicity as a short-term food overdose. You may not react to a food under normal circumstances but if you've eaten it in excess recently, you can become temporarily sensitive to it. This may be more likely to happen if your body is dealing with added stress or other health issues and can often be treated by avoiding the food for a few weeks.

Whether you experience food sensitivities or environmental allergies first, if your immune system is in overdrive attacking one of them, your reaction to the other may get more severe. While your conundrum can seem short-lived, as in the case of seasonal allergies, it might quietly lead to more devastating issues over the long term — like Hashimoto's disease or leaky gut syndrome. Lots of debate and study continue over these disorders, but two great books to read are *Why Do I Still Have Thyroid Symptoms When My Lab Tests Are Normal?* by Datis Kharrazian and *Meals That Heal Inflammation* by Julie Daniluk.

When you suffer from the autoimmune disease **Hashimoto's disease**, also called chronic lymphocytic thyroiditis or autoimmune thyroiditis, your immune system attacks its own cells and organs, including your thyroid gland. As your thyroid gets inflamed, it loses its ability to produce thyroid hormones, which can result in hypothyroidism.

Common symptoms of hypothyroidism include fatigue, constipation, dry skin, increased sensitivity to cold, unexplained weight gain, a puffy face, hoarseness, muscle weakness, elevated blood cholesterol levels, muscles aches, joint pain and/or swelling, irregular periods, thinning hair, slowed heart rate, depression and inhibited memory.

Hashimoto's disease is the most common cause of hypothyroidism in the United States in persons over age 6, according to "Hashimoto Thyroiditis" by Dr. Stephanie Lee on MedScape.com.

But for many reasons, even if you have hypothyroidism, whether related to Hashimoto's disease or not, your lab results can come back normal. And you keep feeling so shoddy.

Meanwhile, for many diagnosed cases of thyroid problems, we pop pills to help our thyroids function better. Sometimes this is necessary. But in many cases, prescription medicines don't truly heal you and don't always continue to work. Well, it's no wonder — if we keep eating foods that our bodies deem enemies the whole time we're "managing" the hypothyroidism!

As your thyroid weakens, you may develop more sensitivities. Your immune system then works even harder to overcome them, and the vicious cycle can put you in a state of feeling unhealthy without being able to detect a cause.

For example, say you have allergies to mold and ragweed. So, you have stuffiness year-round, to some degree. Your body sees gluten as an enemy, but your body doesn't make an obvious response. You keep eating gluten daily. Your immune system is in constant attack mode against the gluten, on top of the mold and ragweed. When does it get a break?

While holistic doctors often advise patients with Hashimoto's disease to remove gluten, gluten may not be the sole culprit. Some research indicates that other seemingly random foods can trigger similar reactions because their molecular content is similar to gluten.

The original list that you may still find online contains several more foods. However, as discussed on thepaleomom.com in "Gluten Cross-Reactivity UPDATE: How your body can still think you're eating gluten even after giving it up," more rigorous research indicates that only the following foods may be true cross-reactors with gluten:

Foods that may cross-react with gluten

some dairy proteins	other
casein	brewer's/baker's yeast
casomorphin	corn
butyrophilin	instant coffee (not fresh coffee)
whey	millet
milk chocolate (due to dairy proteins)	oats
	potato
	rice
	sorghum

The likelihood for cross-reactivity may be related to how sensitive your body is to gluten. For example, if you have celiac disease, you could be sensitive to the cross-reactive foods as well. Even trace amounts of these foods can provoke inflammation or other immune responses.

Sensitivities to the following foods frequently *co-exist* in people with gluten intolerance: amaranth, barley, buckwheat, egg, hemp, Polish wheat, quinoa, rye, sesame, soy, spelt, tapioca, teff and whole milk. But these foods are not true cross-reactors with gluten.

Sadly, your sensitivity to gluten or other foods can go unnoticed for years. Think about it. Many health practitioners advise waiting 72 hours before reintroducing a new food on the elimination diet, used to detect food allergies. Yet it can take 72 hours or longer for your body to react.

Instead, you could reintroduce a new food every 5 to 7 days. But what are the chances in your busy life that within those 5 or 7 days, you have not eaten any other potential culprits, which are quietly compounding your issue but making it difficult to pinpoint blame?

Pay attention to your body's responses and determine what's true for you, knowing your sensitivities may increase or decrease over time depending on many things, including other health conditions, nutrition, stress management and sleep management.

> *This describes what I've experienced. When introducing new foods, I don't notice anything right away. Often, it can take 3 or 4 days to detect stuffiness, and by then I'm not sure if it's from something else I ate, stress, the weather or my period!*
>
> *To top that off, sometimes I notice an itchy throat from some nuts, but not always. I have kept a food journal at times, but to detect the true enemy foods, I would have to introduce one nut or one type of cheese every week.*

Enter the concept of leaky gut. If you don't truly believe it by now, think again. You are what you eat. Your digestive system is like the hub of your mucous membrane network, so everything that goes in to your gut inevitably affects your entire body — even your nose and joints.

If your guts have taken a beating over time from foods that irritate, alcohol or medications (especially antibiotics), they can develop permeations or tiny holes in them. These holes allow food particles to enter your blood stream, essentially infecting your body, because your bloodstream is no place for undigested food. But this "infection" in your body can be quite discrete.

> *As an example, all my lab work has come back normal, but I still encounter occasional moodiness and struggle with chronic congestion. Recently, I've developed food sensitivities and lack energy.*

Think about how all of this corruption can occur in your body because of what you're putting into it, perhaps without knowing it. This is why it's so important to take steps now to feed your body more naturally.

You may think your body tolerates what you're feeding it just fine. But sooner or later, your choices could catch up. Julia Turshen puts it into perfect perspective in *It's All Good* where she explains, "I decided then that my body wasn't an apartment I was renting, it was the house I would always live in."

Whether you have hard-core food allergies or occasionally struggle with a dicey digestive system or sinus issues, this chapter will help you zone in on potential trouble foods (I call them culprits) and provide you with alternatives.

Bear in mind I wrote this book with the notion of using foods as medicine, not *with* medicine. So, always consult your doctor before making drastic changes or substitutions, especially if you have severe food allergies or take prescription medications.

Next, let's get one thing straight. A healthy digestive system should allow you to poop at least once a day, according to my holistic doctors. If you go after every meal, even better. Some doctors say it's OK if you only have one bowel movement (BM) every few days. Well, that might be OK, but if that's your norm, it seems to me that your body is housing whatever you eat way too long — especially if it includes culprit foods.

> It's my opinion that our society today still finds the topic of pooping taboo. Now, in a house with 3 males, frankly, I'm tired of the topic. But you can bet that if my boys haven't been pooping daily, I will change their diet, usually by removing grains and adding water and fruits, and explain to them why. My 4-and 6-year-olds know that water, fruits and veggies help you poop!

eat allergen free

Next time you don't have a healthy bowel movement for a few days, pay attention to how you feel each day. Do you begin to get stuffed up? Bloated? Crabby? Hello! This is NOT normal! It's a sign that your body does not like what you're feeding it.

As your guts react to the foods you eat, they can get irritated and inflamed, in which case your intestinal mucous membrane is reacting to your brain's instruction to "attack" the enemy. And mucous membranes line many other areas of your body, including your nose, mouth, lungs and urinary tract. That's why many diseases and illnesses begin with inflammation somewhere in your body.

Besides Hashimoto's disease and leaky gut syndrome, foods can cause many other more common issues. Of course, sneezing, hives, difficulty swallowing and skin rashes often indicate a food *allergy*. But let's look at a list of common reaction-causing foods, or food culprits, and other symptoms caused by each, whether due to an allergy or sensitivity.

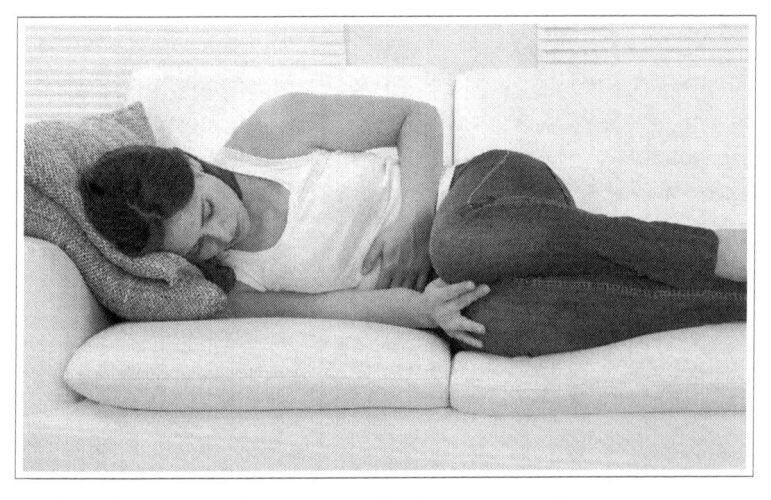

Abdominal issues may include gas, bloating, constipation, nausea or diarrhea.

Common reaction-causing foods and symptoms

Compiled from a variety of sources listed in *Works cited* at the end of this book.

food	symptoms
amines (p. 48)	aggressive behavior especially in kids, depression, eczema, headaches, irritable bowel syndrome
coffee	abdominal issues, difficulty breathing, headaches
dairy	abdominal issues, chronic ear, sinus or chest infections, depression
food colorings (red 1, yellow 5, etc.)	eczema, hyperactivity
gluten, gluten look-alikes (p. 50 and p. 43)	constipation, diarrhea, difficulty concentrating, ADHD, fatigue, infertility, inflamed sinuses/allergies, joint stiffness/arthritis
MSG (monosodium glutamate)	chest pain, feelings of detachment, flushing, headaches, temper tantrums
nightshades, including tomatoes, potatoes, peppers (p. 48)	congestion, inflammation, itchy or watery eyes, joint stiffness, sore throat, shortness of breath
peanuts	chronic bronchitis, irritability, wheezing
pork	abdominal issues, aggression, asthma, difficulty breathing, itchy eyes and nose, sneezing
soy	asthma, bloating, congestion, gas, itchy mouth, personality shift, runny nose
sulfites	abdominal issues, asthma, difficulty concentrating, difficulty swallowing, dizziness, drop in blood pressure, flushing
wheat	abdominal issues, arthritis, asthma, congestion, headaches, nausea, non-stop talking, runny nose

Playing food detective

Amines, formed by the breakdown of proteins in foods, can build up if your body has missing or blocked enzymes. The build-up can result in a sensitivity to that amine. Alcohol, cured meats, eggs, fermented foods, nuts, pork and tomatoes contain a specific amine called tyramine. Avocado and bananas, on the other hand, contain an amine called hydroxytryptamine.

Food additives are countless. But Daniluk offers a simplified list of food additives we should avoid: acesulfame-K, aspartame, butylated hydroxyanisole (BHA), butylated hydroxytoluene (BHT), color dyes FD&C blue 1, 2, green 3, red 3 (erythrosine), red 40, yellow 5 (tartrazine), yellow 6, monosodium glutamate (MSG), parabens, propylene glycol, saccharin, sodium nitrate and sulfites including sulfur dioxide, sodium sulfite, sodium and potassium bisulfate, sodium and potassium melabisulfite and potassium bromate.

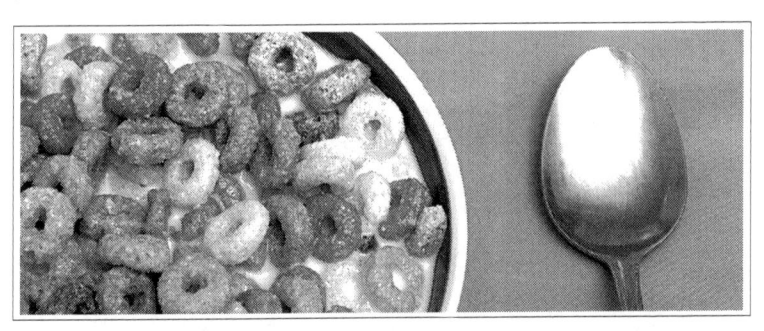

Avoid foods with reds, yellows and blues in the ingredients lists.

Another group, the nightshades, can cause inflammation for some people due to the alkaloid content. Nightshades include cayenne, eggplant, garden huckleberry, ground cherries, hot or sweet peppers, naranjillas, paprika, pepinos, pimentos, potatoes, tamarillos, tomatillos and tomatoes. If you're sensitive to potatoes, tomatoes and bananas, you could be sensitive specifically to the lectin in nightshades and other foods.

If your kids seem hyperactive, act aggressively, have difficulty concentrating or show other symptoms listed in the chart, try eliminating the suspect foods for 3 weeks, under a doctor's advisement to assure proper nutrition. It's a fantastic opportunity to teach your kids how to choose foods responsibly, instead of immediately resorting to medications. You can be supportive by avoiding the foods, too. You might even feel better yourself!

> *One recent year before Thanksgiving, my face blew up to make me look like a battered woman. I realized I had eaten tomatoes or tomato sauce several days in a row and used a new shampoo. After cross-referencing ingredients in my other personal products, I narrowed my suspect to yellow 5. I had my holistic doctor muscle test me for the dye and tomato, and she confirmed I was reacting to both. Since then, I've noticed that not only is yellow 5 in many personal care products — and who cares what color shampoo is? — but in lots of foods as well.*

So, when you notice a strong reaction, stop and assess what you've eaten in the past few days to narrow down your suspects. Remember, it can take 72 hours or more for your body to have a response. Also, if you notice that several foods seem to cause minor discomfort, do a web search like "allergies to tomatoes, bananas and potatoes" to see if they have one common thread. In this case, it's lectin.

If you want to avoid certain foods or categories of foods due to toxicity, intolerance or allergy, use the following chart to make your substitutions easier while still satisfying your taste buds. Note that I have not personally used all of these but have compiled them from many sources as suggestions.

Common reaction-causing foods and substitutes

Compiled from *Simply Gluten Free Magazine, Meals That Heal Inflammation, Let's Eat Out with Celiac/Coeliac & Food Allergies* and personal experiences.

food to avoid	substitute
gluten, found in wheat, rye, barley, bulgur, couscous, durum, einkorn, emmer, farina, faro, graham, matzo, semolina, wheat germ, wheat starch, some caramel color, "stabilizers," flavors, colors, bouillon, many sauces, condiments and soups as a thickening agent, lunchmeats	**flours and starches:** amaranth, arrow root, brown, red or black rice (organic whole grain), buckwheat, cassava, chestnut, corn, Job's tears, millet, nut flours, oats (if certified), potato, quinoa, sorghum, soy, tapioca, taro, teff, yucca **sides:** beans, chickpeas, lentils, peas, potatoes, sweet potatoes
1 egg	1 T ground flax seed + 3 T hot water whisked for 2-3 minutes, then let stand for 5 minutes OR ¼ c applesauce or apricot puree + 2 T oil; add ½ tsp baking powder if baking OR 1 tsp baking powder + 1½ T water + ½ T oil
1 egg white	1 T plain agar powder dissolved in 1 T water; beat, chill for 15 minutes and beat again
1 c casein or dairy	1 c savory broth OR 1 c almond, brown rice or hemp milk for sweetness; add 1 T oil if baking
milk as a drink	brown rice milk, coconut milk, hemp seed milk (non-dairy, casein-free, lactose-free)
1 c milk (full fat)	1 c rice milk + 1 egg yolk OR 1 c water + 1 egg yolk
1 c buttermilk	1 c plain rice or hemp milk + 1 T lemon juice; let stand for 5 minutes to "sour" OR 1 c rice or hemp milk + 1 T apple cider vinegar; let stand for 5 minutes to "sour"

Common reaction-causing foods and substitutes (continued)

food to avoid	substitute
yogurt	unsweetened organic goat or sheep yogurt
1 c butter	1 c coconut butter OR 1 c avocado for cold recipes
salad dressings	unpasteurized apple cider vinegar in a glass bottle (if yeast is not an issue) with lemon or lime juice, garlic and other spices
conventional vinegars	organic, unrefined apple cider, brown rice, fruit, red wine, umeboshi plum vinegars. Avoid conventional balsamic due to the added sugar and note that vinegar is not technically paleo.
1 T fish sauce	1 T tamari sauce, if you can eat soy
1000 mg salmon oil	1 tsp borage seed or algae-based omega-3 oil
½ c ground nuts	½ c coconut flakes OR ½ c ground seeds OR ½ c nut-free granola or crunchy cereal
edamame	whole raw nuts or seeds
1 T miso paste	1 bouillon cube OR 1 tsp umeboshi plum paste
miso soup	fresh vegetable broth
1 c soybeans	¾ c soaked nuts or seeds
1 T tamari	1 T vegetable broth with pinch of salt
tempeh	quinoa and black beans

Common reaction-causing foods and substitutes

(continued from p. 51)

food to avoid	substitute
starches/legumes: alfalfa, beans, carob, chickpeas, clover, lentils, lupines, mesquite, peanuts, peas, potatoes, soybeans, tamarind, wisteria, etc.	cauliflower (great for hummus), raw or cooked kohlrabi, sweet potatoes, squash

Kohlrabi can be eaten raw like a radish, sautéed like fries or prepared many other ways, although it's not always in season or easy to find. Use the leaves for your lunchmeat wraps sans bread.

chips, snack bars, crackers	flavored nori seaweed without MSG or sugar, fresh fruit, gluten-free organic beef jerky, hard-boiled eggs, homemade chips (organic kale, apple, sweet potato, dulce or beet), nuts or seeds (pumpkin and sunflower), organic, gluten-free lunch meat slices, raw veggies such as celery, carrot, cucumber, zucchini or bell peppers, with nut butter or hummus, if desired
1 c refined white or brown cane sugar	1 c coconut palm sugar
1 c corn syrup	1 c honey OR 1 c agave nectar OR 1 c maple syrup
milk chocolate	dark chocolate with at least 70% cacao and cocoa butter but *without* hydrogenated oils, additives and added sugar

Both milk and dark chocolate contain flavonoids, which act as antioxidants. But milk chocolate contains milk and therefore fewer flavonoids, plus added sugar. Milk also is thought to bind with flavonoids, making them unavailable and reducing the health benefits of the chocolate. So, choose dark chocolate, and if you're eating it for antioxidant effects, avoid drinking milk with it.

Going gluten free

A friend of mine innocently and understandably posed a question as to whether people eating gluten free or grain free actually feel better because they're avoiding those ingredients, or because they're eating more vegetables, fruits and lean proteins. This is a valid argument. But it's not one I've tested because when I remove gluten, *I have* to add something! Gluten and grains are what we Americans rely on so heavily to fill us up. So, if you could only remove the gluten from your diet and make no other changes, you might get your answer. Or, you can remove the gluten while working with your doctor to make sure you're getting proper nutrition. If you feel better as a result, isn't that your end goal anyhow?

Going gluten free seems to be widespread. Whether you're doing it as a cleanse or permanently, eating gluten free is a bit of an art for many of us bread and carb fanatics!

First, make sure product labels say "GF," "gluten-free," "no gluten," "free of gluten" or "without gluten," indicating that they follow the FDA regulation of containing less than 20 parts per million (ppm) of gluten. Otherwise, for example, corn or oat products may not contain gluten, but may be processed on equipment used for other gluten-containing products. This is called cross-contamination.

Buy foods labeled "gluten-free" in moderation, though, because they are often made from brown rice or potato flour, which are gluten look-alikes (p. 43) that also could bother you. Brown rice is difficult for some people to digest, and potatoes are a nightshade, which can cause inflammation. Also note that many gluten-free products still have other harmful additives or GMOs, unless they are organic *and* gluten free.

Instead of buying more packaged gluten-free foods, replace grains and starches with vegetables when possible. Consider:

- kohlrabi instead of potatoes.
- zucchini or sweet potato slices instead of buns.
- veggie medley instead of rice.

The easiest way to go gluten free is to substitute fresh foods. Otherwise, you need to plan on spending lots of time reading labels and recognizing other terms for gluten. Consider using a modified paleo plan to get used to eating fresh and then add back some foods you tolerate that are not paleo.

Eating gluten free in our bread-loving country takes some trial, error and patience. Here are a few more specific tips to help you get started.

1. Focus on eating whole fresh foods, including fruits, vegetables, fresh meats but not deli meats or packaged meats, unless you know they are GF.

2. For breakfast, consider eggs, GF sausage or bacon without nitrates, sweet potatoes, GF granola, yogurt and fruit or nuts.

3. For lunch, use large leaf lettuce to wrap your now breadless sandwich. Eat more salads with GF dressing or homemade soups without gluten. Leftovers are a great option, too.

4. Rely on cut raw veggies with hummus, nuts and fruits for snacks.

5. Cook a lean meat or fish with roasted or sautéed vegetables for dinner. Use sweet potato or zucchini slices as your bun for burger night.

6. Buy gluten-free flour with xanthan gum and substitute this for regular flour when making desserts. They may not be as fluffy as usual, but neither will your guts, perhaps.

7. Use gluten-free bread, chips or breakfast items sparingly to help your transition, because they could contain corn, rice, potato or other grains that can cause inflammation.

8. Search online as more people go gluten free and share recipes or ideas for making it easier.

9. If eating out, ask if a menu item is gluten free, especially if you have celiac. You don't want any rude surprises!

10. Be bold about it. Don't feel ashamed or be hesitant to ask for GF. Think of it as a way to educate the rest of society about eating healthier, too!

For kids in school, going gluten free can be difficult. I suggest telling staff members that your kid needs to avoid gluten, even if it's only a sensitivity, packing all his food and educating him about why he can't eat it. You can find all kinds of lunch ideas online by searching for gluten-free or paleo lunches for kids.

Just as substituting gluten-free products for gluten can backfire, so can subbing unsweetened almond milk for milk. Almond milk is better used as a condiment or for baking rather than as a staple drink, because almonds have a high level of omega-6 fatty acids. A diet high in omega-6 and without enough omega-3 can increase inflammation.

Finally, note that when you give up your food allergen or food culprit, you might experience withdrawal symptoms, similar to the allergy symptoms on p. 47, *at first*. This is a good indicator that you need to give it up for a while, and these symptoms should subside soon.

No matter what subs you choose, be sure to consult with your doctor first if you have other health conditions. Rotate substitutes daily to avoid developing new sensitivities. All things in moderation is best.

With these substitution ideas, hopefully you can fulfill any cravings without missing your culprit food! If you're worried about not getting enough of a certain nutrient when you have to avoid a healthy food, reference this chart for other sources of that nutrient that you may digest more easily.

The nutrients you need and common food sources

Extracted from *101 Natural Healthy Eating Tips* by Emily Davidson as well as various online sources and personal experience.

nutrient	source
calcium builds stronger bone, maintains heart, muscle and nerve function	fish, leafy greens, nuts, organic dairy, sea vegetables, sesame seeds, spinach
electrolytes maintain blood chemistry, blood pressure, nerve function and muscle function, hydrate and rebuild damaged tissue	coconut water
fiber prevents constipation and maintains healthy weight	apples or pears with skin, artichokes, beans, berries, broccoli, brown rice, Brussels sprouts, carrots, nuts (primarily almonds, pecans and walnuts), peas, turnips
iodine supports proper thyroid function and proper development of skeletal and central nervous systems in fetuses and infants	kelp, nori, salt-water fish and seafood, vegetables grown in soil with adequate levels of iodine
iron boosts your immune system and energy while distributing oxygen to your organs	chickpeas, lentils, pumpkin seeds, sesame seeds, soybeans, spinach
magnesium relaxes your nerves and muscles while strengthening your bones	black beans, pumpkin seeds, sesame seeds, spinach, Swiss chard

Note that this is not a complete list of nutrients, functions or sources but is intended for use as a guide as you consult with your doctor, make adjustments to your diet and strive for optimal nutrition.

The nutrients you need and common food sources (continued)	
nutrient	**source**
omega-3 fats reduce inflammation and help keep your arteries from thickening while increasing brain function and regulating your mood	some algae, eggs, (mainly in yolks, especially in enriched), fresh-caught cold-water fish such as salmon, ocean krill, seeds (flax, chia, perilla, sacha inchi), walnuts, winter squash including acorn, butternut, hubbard, kabocha, pumpkin, turban
potassium maintains blood flow and heart function	avocados, bananas, coconut water, oranges, spinach, strawberries, tomatoes
probiotics help balance flora to improve intestinal health while boosting immune function	some aged cheese including cheddar, Gouda, parmesan and Swiss, Amazake rice, kefir, kimchi*, kombucha drinks, miso including soy and red bean if you tolerate soy, rakfish, sauerkraut*, Sicilian green olives*, sourdough from whole grain flour, taro root; yogurt without sugar substitutes *vinegar-free, fermented versions
sodium helps regulate water balance while controlling muscle and nerve function and supporting the circulatory system	celery, kelp, lean meats, nori, salt-water fish and seafood, spinach
vitamin D aids absorption of calcium for healthy bones, reduces blood pressure and boosts immune function	eggs, mackerel, milk (from cows, goats or sheep), salmon, tuna

A note about caffeine (not a nutrient but just being real!)

Instead of drinking coffee or soda, consider drinking smoky-flavored yerba mate tea. Neither a green nor black tea, yerba mate tea is believed to promote more steady energy without giving you the jitters. It's also credited for weight loss, colon cleansing, accelerated healing, stress relief and allergy control. But even it has controversy surrounding it, so read up and drink it in moderation if at all.

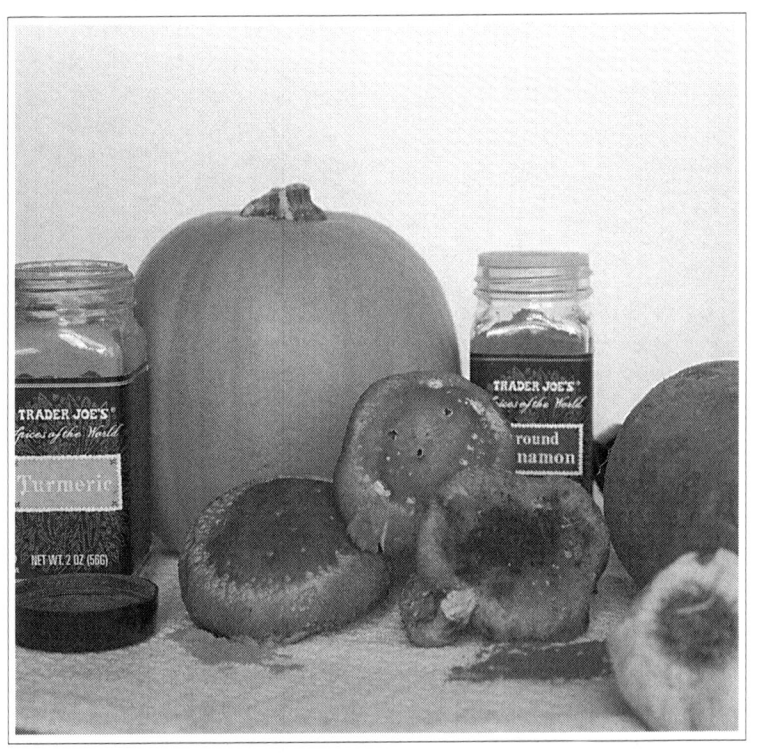

Learn to use foods for their natural medicinal effects.

If you want to enlist foods specifically for medicinal purposes, add these delish items to your diet (list compiled from Julie

Daniluk's *Meals That Heal Inflammation*, personal learning and online sources about spices).

Garlic boosts your immune system by increasing white blood cell production and helping to extract carcinogens and other toxins.

Papaya provides substantial vitamin C, which helps absorb iron and serves as an antihistamine while increasing white blood cells and antibody production. You can get vitamin C from bell peppers, broccoli, Brussels sprouts, cauliflower, kale, raspberries and strawberries.

Shiitake mushrooms provide lentinan, which boosts your immunity.

Sesame seeds are rich in zinc, which helps increase your fighting T-cells, and plant sterols, which help prevent autoimmune disorders and cancer while lowering cholesterol.

Squash, pumpkins and sweet potatoes provide beta-carotene, which your body converts to vitamin A, to repair lung cells and boost your infection-fighting cells.

Spices offer countless health benefits, too. Fresh is best. Just a few examples: **Cayenne pepper** boosts immune function and revs metabolism, though it is a nightshade. **Cinnamon** is thought to reduce inflammation and blood sugar while warding off illness and making anything yummier. **Turmeric** is an Indian flavoring that reduces inflammation and protects against cancer. A little goes a long way!

As you identify your culprit foods, take a break from them and let your body heal, you may eventually add them back in moderation, though this may not be as successful if you have a food *allergy*. Be aware that you could, however, become more sensitive to that food.

> *Even if you choose not to identify your food enemies, you can still use these lists to troubleshoot. For example, in my household, if we're not pooping daily, we remove gluten and/or other grains and insert fruits, vegetables and more water. When I feel crabby, I reduce my already moderate intake of gluten for a few days. And as an anti-inflammatory, I drink a cup of tea with cinnamon, turmeric and raw honey.*

Using foods medicinally and eating preventively may take several months to get used to, but you *can* get used to it. And eating more naturally will become second nature and more enjoyable.

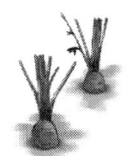

7. take a paleo-like plunge

If you want to eat natural to the max, consider a paleo or paleo-like diet. But acknowledge a few important realities first.

1. In the long-term, this is not really a diet but a change in lifestyle, and a rather demanding one — of your self-discipline, time and effort to plan, prepare and cook.

2. A *paleo diet* can be done for 2-3 weeks as a cleansing diet. Your liver should filter out toxins on its own. But if it's been overloaded with alcohol, prescription or other drugs, or foods you didn't even know were irritants, your liver might need a little "vaca" time to unwind. Added stress or sickness can overwork your liver, too.

3. Whether you're considering the paleo diet as a cleanse or lifestyle change, I suggest consulting with your doctor first, so you don't inadvertently make any medical condition worse, like eating too much fruit if you're diabetic.

Now, let's get into the good stuff. What is a paleo-like food plan?

A paleo diet embraces a palette of grass-produced meats, eggs, fish and seafood, fresh fruits and vegetables, seeds and nuts as well as healthy oils. Whenever possible, opt for organic products with no GMOs. You should avoid grains, corns or potatoes (except sweet potatoes with orange insides), legumes (including peanuts), dairy, processed foods, refined sugars and vegetable oils. With possibly a few exceptions, you will nix liquor consumption, too.

Put simply, it's hard core. You can modify a paleo plan as you and your doctor see fit and still reap many health benefits from it. But the paleo-like plan I'm presenting goes pretty extreme so you get the true picture.

Paleo-like food plan

Meats

Eat fresh caught wild fish, lean organic meats and eggs, all in moderation. Choose meats, deli meats and sausages that have been grass-fed or pasture-raised with no additives and minimal nitrates.

Vegetables

Opt for organic vegetables. Note that corn and potatoes are not considered vegetables but starches. Instead, choose only sweet potatoes that are orange on the inside but not every day if they make you feel sluggish or if they make it difficult to lose weight.

Fruits

Eat organic fruits in moderation.

Nuts and seeds

Choose organic, raw nuts, nut butters and seeds. If watching your weight, opt for lower calorie nuts such as almonds, cashews and pistachios. Use various nut or seed butters — almond, sunflower, cashew and more — as dips or spreads.

Oils and butter

Your best choices are avocado oil for high-heat cooking and organic extra virgin olive oil for low heat. Cooking oils on higher heat than recommended can make them rancid and toxic. If you eat a modified paleo diet and use butter, then choose organic, grass-fed products or organic, clarified ghee, which doesn't contain lactose or casein. Remember, though, that both are considered dairy since they're made from milk.

Spices

Experiment with more beneficial spices to create unique flavors for your food. Use Himalayan crystal salt in moderation. Sodium can be good for hydration, especially for athletes, but too much can stress out your kidneys or worsen congestive heart failure. A spritz of lemon juice makes a great salt alternative, as it naturally amplifies flavor similarly to salt.

Alcohol

Any alcohol technically violates the paleo diet. But I want to keep it realistic here. If you desire an occasional drink, consider gluten-free wine or gluten-free vodka over ice, sans the sugary mixers.

So, AVOID:

- all grains, especially wheat and gluten but also rice and corn.
- dairy.
- legumes and starchy vegetables, including alfalfa, beans, carob, chickpeas, clover, lentils, lupines, mesquite, peanuts, peas, potatoes, soybeans, tamarind and wisteria.
- refined sugars.
- processed foods.
- additives and chemicals — if a food contains an ingredient you can't pronounce, don't buy it.

Sarah Fragoso noted in *Everyday Paleo* that gluten may be your worst form of cheating because it can take up to 15 days to recover from 1 dose, the equivalent of 1 piece of toast or 1 beer. Some sources say it can take several months to recover from 1 dose of gluten. It will likely vary based on factors like your body's tolerance of it, other health issues, stress, etc.

So, how does eating paleo look day to day?

- Most likely, you will need to eat several small meals each day to feel satisfied or full, at least until your body adjusts to the lack of starches and grains. It's important not to skip breakfast, and you may find it helpful to eat it before 7:30 a.m., which seemed to help sustain my energy level.
- Breakfast may no longer look like breakfast. It may look more like dinner. Be open-minded.
- Grains are evil on this plan. Embrace creativity in the kitchen.

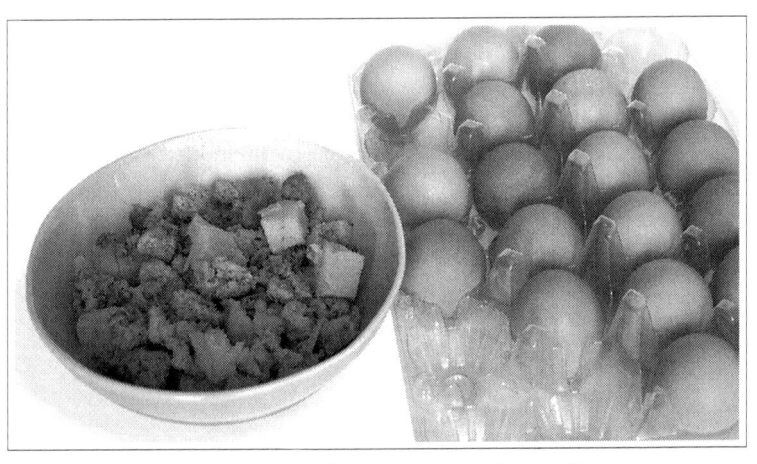

Substitute sweet potatoes, paleo sausage and eggs for your traditional breakfast.

Before deeming your house a paleo-like abode, consider easing into it so you have a few weeks to adapt to shopping, planning and preparing meals ahead of time. Microwaving foods isn't ideal. But unless one parent stays at home or only works part-time, cooking all meals fresh can be frustrating. Consider shopping ahead instead and choosing 2 nights per week — Sunday and Wednesday, for example — to grill meats and prepare other sides that may take longer to make.

Also, find some go-to foods and keep them on hand, so it's easier to stick to your paleo plan. Here are some examples.

Breakfast: hard-boiled eggs, frozen fruit, nuts, seeds

Lunch: gluten-free lunchmeat wrapped in large lettuce leaves or paleo-style chicken salad

Snack: dried fruit without added sugars or added fruit concentrate, raw fruits and veggies, gluten-free beef jerky with minimal nitrates, nuts, plantain chips with guacamole, seeds

Dinner: lean organic meat or fish, grilled or sautéed veggies

When eating out, choose:

- to hold the gluten, including croutons, cheese and other dressings or sauces.
- grilled chicken or hamburger sans the bun.
- double veggies instead of fries, potatoes or rice.
- olive oil, lemon and pepper or salsa instead of pre-made salad dressings.
- fajitas with guacamole but without rice, beans and tortillas for Mexican.
- curry dishes without soy sauce and with veggies instead of rice for Thai.

To help you get started, you can find several paleo meal plans online, or you can reference the one in chapter 10.

Perhaps you already eat like a health nut and going paleo is not that drastic for you. Good for you and congrats! Your body thanks you.

> However, for me, eating paleo-like on the Repairvite diet was a cleanse — on one month, off one, then on again — and a major undertaking as I love to eat and have a beer. Also, I enjoy cooking and getting creative in the kitchen but don't want to make it my full-time job. And shopping ranks up there with cleaning as a necessary evil.
>
> Next, I can practically out-eat my husband and when I remove grains, it's hard for me to feel full or even satisfied. And by satisfied, I mean not hungry and bitchy! I didn't see earth-shattering results. I don't get so congested now that I can't breathe or talk like a normal human being. But my immune system is not where it should be.
>
> Still, I've learned how to incorporate many new foods into my diet, which makes eating things in moderation easier. Plus, eating more naturally on a day-to-day basis has become my new norm. I believe this helps to minimize my body's unnecessary attacks, so that my immune system is not as taxed.
>
> I can teach what I've learned to my kids so they can begin eating healthy now at young ages, respect how foods can help or harm and be better equipped to make informed choices as they grow more independent.

If we teach our kids how to make healthier choices and why this is so important, they have a better chance to live healthier than our own generation. We can even instill healthier eating from our baby's day one, which we'll cover next.

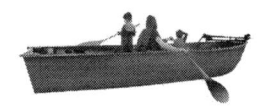

8. feed your baby more naturally

Doctors' recommendations on how to start your baby onto solid foods have changed drastically, even since my firstborn came along. I've heard from the more traditional "start cereals as early as 4 months but avoid some foods that are more common allergens" to "have your baby try almost every food pureed before age 1" as a way to help prevent food allergies. Theories are likely to keep changing.

So, what's really best?

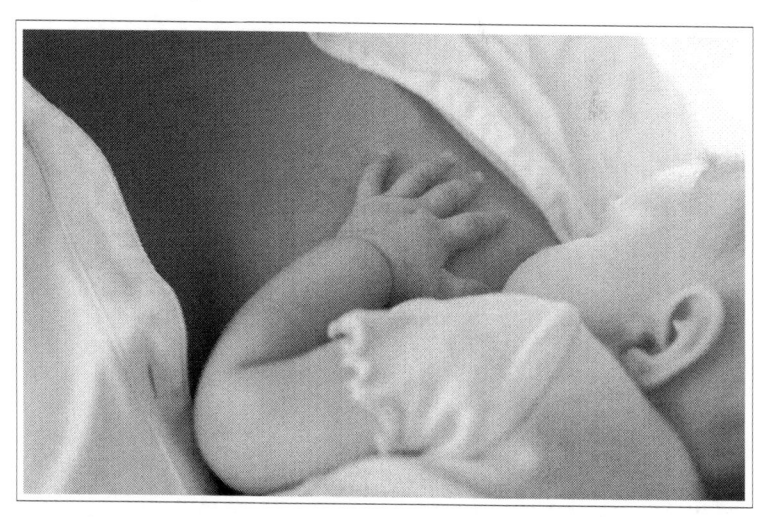

Breastfeeding provides your baby with loads of nutrients and helps build her immune system naturally.

I'm no doctor or pediatrician, and I haven't fed my kids perfectly by a long shot. It gets even harder to do when they go to daycare and school, where they are subjected to a high-carb diet with plenty of GMOs. But one holistic doctor has seen my family through several years of unraveling my own toxicities. She has also seen my kids through the immunizations I dread and thankfully only a few minor illnesses. I fully trust her theory on how to feed babies, and it makes the most sense to me. So, let me sum up suggestions about how to start your baby on solids from Laurie Berger, doctor of chiropractic.

1. Breastfeed for at least 1 year.

2. Grains: Have you seen what happens to baby cereal after it sits out for 10 minutes? That's what it's doing in your baby's tummy, too. Grains are not easy to digest and can magnify congestion or ear infections. Skip the grains at first.

3. Give him a probiotic powder for infants to promote a balance of yeasts and bacteria that will help his digestive system mature — about ¼ teaspoon daily on the breast or in bottled breast milk, and later mixed in foods.

4. When starting solids, start with root vegetables because they are easier to digest. Some good choices include carrots, beets, parsnips, rutabagas, squash, sweet potatoes and turnips. Wait 3 days or longer before introducing any new foods, so you can detect allergic symptoms or other reactions.

5. Introduce purified water instead of milk in a sippy cup.

6. Add easy-to-digest pears and apples before progressing to other fruits. Know that avocados are rich in nutrients while bananas can be binding.

7. At 1 year, *gradually* add in soft cheeses, such as ricotta and cottage.

8 Introduce *gradually* a variety of 100% whole grains, and watch for any reactions, including aggressive behavior or gassiness — not just bumps or itchiness.

9 Meats can wait, especially if he's eating adequate greens, beans or eggs.

10 Avoid honey, nuts and strawberries till about age 2.

With a proper mix of these foods, you shouldn't have to subject him to over-processed milk, cow, soy or otherwise, to obtain proper nutrition.

> *When I had my first child, I didn't yet know about Dr. Berger's recommendations. I started him on cereals around 4 months, and he had issues with ear infections for a few months. When we visited Dr. Berger, she recommended taking cereals out of his diet and focusing on easily digested veggies and fruits instead. His ear infections cleared up, and he has not had ear issues since.*
>
> *With my second son, I skipped grains until he was 9 months, then used them sparingly, usually in the form of organic veggie puffs. He has never had an ear infection. It could be coincidence, but I tend to think not!*

The idea behind Dr. Berger's plan is to feed your baby what his developing body can handle as it matures. You can help his system to mature at a natural pace instead of pushing it to develop faster and potentially overtaxing it.

Ultimately, you need to do what you feel is best, but this can serve as a guideline to helping your baby eat more naturally while you do, too.

Now, let's talk shopping to make your mission of eating more naturally easier — whether you're taking baby steps or the paleo-like plunge.

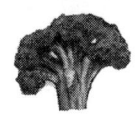

9. shop smarter

In this chapter, we'll discuss how to shop for a paleo-like plunge. You can always scale back your efforts if you'd rather just eat greener grub or avoid food allergens and culprits.

Plan on shopping at least twice per week, unless you can buy some unripened produce that will hold longer. Consider health food stores, such as Trader Joe's or Whole Foods for more organic options. You'll primarily shop a store's perimeter, the outermost aisles with fresh foods. You may buy some canned or frozen goods, but they should not contain additives or anything you can't recognize!

What to look for on the labels

Produce

- Buy 100% certified organic fruits and vegetables to avoid pesticides or fertilizers. Avocadoes, cantaloupes, grapefruit, kiwi, mangoes, pineapple, watermelon, asparagus, cabbage, eggplant, mushrooms, onions and sweet potatoes tend to have less exposure to pesticides.

- Because Asian mushrooms are grown on wood or tree stumps, they are safer than portabellas or button mushrooms, which usually grow on manure.

- Make an effort to find organic dried fruit, since it cannot be washed, with no added sugar, juice concentrate or sugar substitutes.

- When you buy canned, opt for organic items with minimal ingredients, such as green beans with only sea salt added.

Nuts and seeds (except peanuts)
- When buying nuts and seeds, opt for raw, dry-roasted and unsalted versions, because chopped or presliced nuts are more likely to contain damaged oils. If you eat peanuts, part of the legume family, on a modified paleo plan, do so

Paleo shopping list — pantry (organic ideally)

canned	dried
diced tomatoes (no salt added)	coconut flakes (refrigerate after opening)
tomato paste	coconut flour
jalapenos	almond flour or meal
diced green chiles	dried unsweetened Bing cherries
olives	dried unsweetened figs
artichoke hearts	dried unsweetened apricots
apple cider vinegar, ideal for oil and vinegar dressing	unsweetened plantain chips
almond butter or sunflower butter	beef jerky (gluten-free and soy-free)
tahini paste	sun-dried tomatoes
free-range, gluten-free chicken broth	spices (including Pink Himalayan salt)
wild-caught Alaskan salmon	
tuna	

nuts	oils
raw almonds	avocado oil
raw pecans	coconut oil
raw walnuts	olive oil

sparingly as they tend to be high in inflammation-causing molds. Remember that almonds offer many nutrients such as vitamin E, magnesium and potassium, but also contain a high level of omega-6s. If your omega-6 content is high already, eat almond products sparingly, if at all.

- Sprouted or soaked seeds are easier to digest.
- Consider using organic tahini paste that contains only sesame seeds for dressings, marinades or hummus.

Paleo shopping list — refrigerator (organic ideally)

fresh fruits and veggies	condiments
(not corn, legumes or potatoes) carrots cucumber kale lettuce spinach squash sweet potatoes (orange inside) apples blueberries lemons limes pears strawberries	(gluten-free versions) hot sauce salsa Thai fish oil Thai curry paste fermented sauerkraut mustard plain unsweetened almond milk
meats	**drinks**
eggs (free-range or omega-3 enriched, soy-free) deli meat (nitrate-free and gluten-free) free-range chicken grass-fed ground beef	coconut water unsweetened coconut milk

Oils

Select organic, unrefined, cold-pressed oils instead of expeller-pressed oils. Use them within a year or throw them out. And be sure to cook only at the recommended heat level to avoid making them rancid.

- for dressings: extra virgin olive oil
- for sautéing: coconut oil, virgin olive oil
- for high-heat cooking: avocado oil, grape seed oil, sunflower oil or light olive oil (light refers to color and taste)

A note about product labels

Read health claims on packaged goods carefully. As we've learned, "whole grain" doesn't mean organic or even 100% whole grain. And "100% of your daily vitamin C" does not necessarily make a juice healthy. It could still contain too much sugar, sugar substitutes or corn syrup.

Before shopping, you may want to review chapter 4 for guidance about reading labels. Also, you can find information about the purity and safety of products at ewg.org (Environmental Working Group).

Next, let's cook up a plan.

10. plan and prepare healthier meals

With a little meal planning, eating more naturally will feel more feasible. By tweaking your meal preparation, you can make even bigger strides in eating healthier. And every step you take to eat more organically could help remove a little layer of toxicity from your life.

Plan

Maybe you prefer to throw dinner together each night, depending on what you have and crave. That's perfectly fine. But if the nightly mystery of "What are we going to do for dinner tonight?" deflates you like it does my husband and me, a little meal planning can make preparation easier. And like everything else, you can take meal planning to various extremes.

1. You can move foods from the freezer to the fridge to thaw on Sunday night and have an idea of what you're going to cook that week.

2. You can have a vague menu for dinner each night of the week.

3. You can prepare a full-blown menu for the week or month and stick to it religiously.

> *While I was doing the paleo-like Repairvite cleansing diet for 2 months, I used a 2-week menu for reference, especially to help during my brain-dead and starved moments. Now, I loosely stick to method #1, because I like to keep things fluid and flexible. Plus, my appetite has leveled off a bit, so I'm not feeling as ravenous 24/7.*

Figuring out which meal planning method helps you the most could take trial and error. You will find countless ideas for paleo meals online, from simple to extravagant. Because we are so busy and many of us would rather spend more time with the kids than in the kitchen, let's look at some rather simple ideas for a paleo meal plan.

Paleo meal plan

"Paleo" indicates you need to be sure to use paleo recipes (chicken salad without mayonnaise). This plan does not include spices, but you should add whatever spices you like.

	Monday	Tuesday	Wednesday
breakfast	sweet potato boats stuffed with paleo sausage	eggs with paleo bacon	broccoli and tomato frittata
lunch	turkey, guacamole and lettuce wraps with olives and cucumbers	leftovers from dinner	paleo chicken or vegetable soup with kohlrabi fries
snack	apple slices with almond butter	paleo snack bars	raw veggies with cauliflower hummus
dinner	grilled chicken and broccoli	grilled lemon cod with asparagus	hamburgers and sautéed Swiss chard

Remember that you may want to grill food for a couple of nights at one time. Also, these are ideas based on what I've found that's tasty and/or simple. This has not been reviewed by a nutritionist for daily vitamin, mineral or caloric intake. But even if you're not going full-blown paleo, this will help you convert some of your snacks and meals. Be open-minded and creative!

Generally, the fewer items in a meal, the easier it will be to digest. According to Geoff Bond in *Natural Eating, Natural Anthropology*, at least 40% of your diet should be hardy vegetables, with 25% of it being fruits. He adds that veggies are best digested with proteins or starches and that fruits are best digested when eaten solo.

Consider other proteins and vegetables, such as shrimp, scallops, veal, lamb, Brussels sprouts, cabbage and many others. If you insist on a "bun" for your burger, use grilled sweet potato or zucchini slices.

Thursday	Friday	Saturday	Sunday
kohlrabi cakes and paleo sausage	bacon and spinach omelet	paleo chicken wings and paleo pumpkin biscuits	mixed nuts, sweet potato muffins and fresh fruit
lettuce salad with grilled chicken or tuna and sweet potato chips	grilled chicken fingers and veggies with cauliflower hummus	paleo chicken salad and paleo cauliflower with leek soup	paleo sausage with sauerkraut
mixed berries or other fresh fruit with nuts	plantain chips with guacamole	sweet potato and beet chips	paleo banana muffins
sliced flank steak with kohlrabi fries	grilled salmon, lettuce salad and grilled sweet potatoes	zucchini noodles with tomato sauce and spinach salad	paleo barbecued turkey legs and sautéed kale with red onion

plan and prepare healthier meals

Bond advises *not* to eat:

- starches with fruit or protein, which rules out our beloved meat-and-potatoes meal.
- proteins with starches.
- proteins with fruits.

So, veggies are the best side for proteins. The good news is that sweet potatoes are considered a veggie rather than a starch and can help paleo eaters feel more full.

Remember, other potatoes are not allowed on the paleo diet, as they are starches — and a member of the nightshade family, in case those bother you. Besides, because the potato is not highly nutritious despite its potassium, Bond considers it a bad carb. He suggests eating only a few steamed or boiled potatoes with no other bad carbs if you insist on eating them.

Prepare

You can also make healthier choices about how you prepare meals.

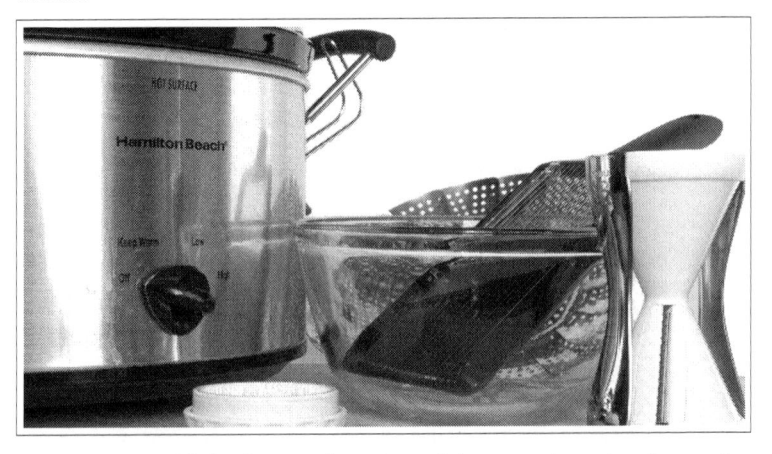

Get creative with kitchen tools — in stainless steel or glass instead of plastic whenever possible.

Tools and cookware

- Avoid plastic. When combined with heat from a dishwasher or heated food, chemicals such as BPA or phthalates can migrate into the foods you eat. These chemicals can mimic, change or shut down your body's chemical signals that regulate metabolism, reproduction and response to stress. They can be detrimental especially during critical times of development, according to webmd.com, such as when a fetus' brain or sex organs are developing in the womb.

  Now, health experts are questioning the safety of BPA-free plastics too, due to the chemicals they contain.

- Choose glass containers at home and use stainless steel containers for your kids' lunchboxes and water bottles.

- Select stainless steel, cast iron, glass, titanium or enamel-coated cookware instead of nonstick ware, which often contains estrogen-mimicking chemicals that could be linked to hormone imbalance and even infertility.

- Opt for wooden cutting boards instead of plastic for the same reason.

- Make sure you have a sharp set of knives and a steam basket.

- Mandolin slicers and spiral vegetable slicers add variety of texture.

- Use an oil mister to coat your veggies lightly before cooking them.

- You may also enjoy the convenience of a food processor, blender or juicer, unless you prefer chewing as a means to feel fuller.

- If you want to save time, consider purchasing a pressure cooker or slow cooker (crockpot) for meats, beans, veggies, soups and more.

Washing foods

Wash your fruits and vegetables with a vinegar and water solution or similar product just before you eat them. Otherwise, they may mold more quickly. If you wash them ahead, add a paper towel to the container to collect moisture, then remove it the next morning. Consider flipping containers of fresh fruits or lettuce every other day or so to aerate them and help delay molding.

Always wash canned goods, since metals may contain toxins like BPA or phthalates. Have you ever noticed how canned beans suds up when you rinse them? Wash, rinse and repeat!

Cooking with oils

Cook with oils at their recommended heat levels to avoid making them rancid.

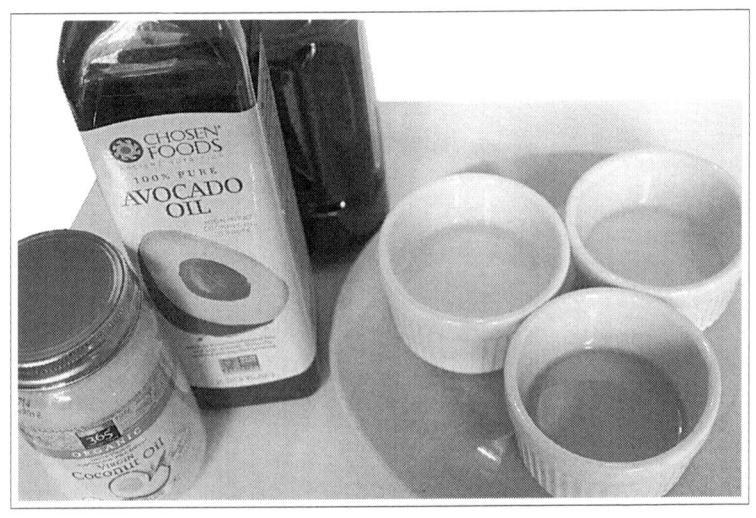

Cook with organic, unrefined cold-pressed oils at appropriate temperatures to avoid making them rancid and potentially harmful.

Cooking with oil guide

Extracted from clevelandclinic.org and organicauthority.com.

oil	approximate smoke point	notes
high heat oils for searing or browning		
almond	430°	nutty flavor
avocado	520°	sweet aroma
medium-high heat oils for baking, cooking or stir-frying		
extra virgin olive	375°	best oil overall; refined and light
grape seed	420°	high in omega-6
medium heat oils for light sautéing, low-heat baking and sauces		
coconut	350°	moderate use; high in saturated fat
hemp	330°	good source of omega-3s; keep refrigerated
no heat oils for dips, dressings or marinades		
extra virgin olive	375°	best oil overall; refined and light
flaxseed	225°	good source of alpha-linolenic acid, an omega-3

Microwaving

If you're trying to limit exposure to radiation, avoid using the microwave … and your laptop, cell phone or other electronic devices, for that matter, according to "To Nuke or Not to Nuke? Should You Microwave Your Food?" from *The Oz Blog*.

> *Even if I was not working, I would not want to spend the bulk of my time shopping and cooking every meal from scratch, especially on busy evenings between school, a couple of kids' practices and their early bedtime. So, call me busted. I use the microwave. How bad am I for using it, anyway?*

Microwaving food may not be ideal for your health, but by using these tips from *The Oz Blog's* article, you can help minimize the ill effects from it.

- Make sure that your microwave has no cracks or gaps and that the door is hinged properly.
- Use high-quality fresh or frozen foods in microwave-safe, BPA-free containers.
- Use minimal water and cooking time to preserve nutrients.
- Stand *several feet* away from the microwave while cooking.

Eat and enjoy

Use these suggestions to eat smarter, digest more easily and truly enjoy.

- Eat vegetables first. Despite the trend to puree or juice everything, chewing actually helps you feel full and satisfied, so that's a matter of preference. You may also want to blend veggies into your kids' food if they haven't developed a taste for them, although it's a better idea to help them develop that taste. It may take up to 10 times of *seeing* a new food before a child will even try it, according to "Open Your Mind (and Your Mouth) to New Foods" on webmd.com. So, stand strong and offer frequently even as your stubborn child declines the healthier foods. Don't give up!

- If you aren't eating paleo and *do* eat grains, try replacing 1 or 2 servings a day with vegetables. For breakfast, consider eggs and sweet potato hash instead of eggs and toast. For a snack, eat raw veggie sticks instead of crackers and cheese.
- Eat at consistent times each day, in a low-stress, quiet environment.
- Chew thoroughly until you can identify a food by its taste only and not its texture.
- Sip warm or room temperature liquids rather than cold ones, particularly if you have health issues related to digestion. The theory is that your body will use its energy to help warm the cold liquids instead of using its energy to help digest your food.
- Allow your meal to last longer so you can eat slower. Eating healthy meals together as a family will reinforce good eating habits, too.
- Sit with good posture.
- Stop eating before you feel full.
- Avoid heavy meals 2 to 3 hours before bedtime.
- Whether you plan a lot or a little, always make sure you have items to eat on hand, so you don't sabotage your natural eating to stave off hunger pains and potential bitchiness!
- Replace utensils and tools, so your food preparation compliments your new natural eating habits. While you're at it, educate your kids about why you are making these changes.

- Get creative. Go online and search for "recipes using xyz without abc" for fresh ideas.

- Experiment and have fun cooking with your spouse or kids. Try using a spiral cutter to make noodles out of squash instead of wheat flour or another gluten-containing grain. Smell up your entire house when you make your own apple cinnamon chips. Have you dared to dabble with kohlrabi?! Eat it raw. Use it to make fries or use the huge leaves for a wrap. And then there's cauliflower hummus for the starch intolerant.

It's time to eat so you can enjoy a happier, healthier life. It's your right and your opportunity to change the way you feel. I hope now that you're encouraged to savor the journey, too.

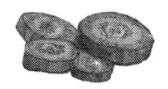

11. you may not be excused

If you're still feeling skeptical about eating healthier, keep reading!

Over the years, I've spewed out many reasons why I couldn't eat healthier or avoid gluten. I love beer, after all! I've heard many reasons from others, too. But when you get down to it, they are all just excuses. If you're really determined to eat healthier — if you have to avoid something due to allergic reactions or if you just want to be around longer for your children — you can and will find ways to make it happen.

Start by acknowledging some seemingly valid arguments, reasons, excuses or whatever you wish to call them, and my rebuttals.

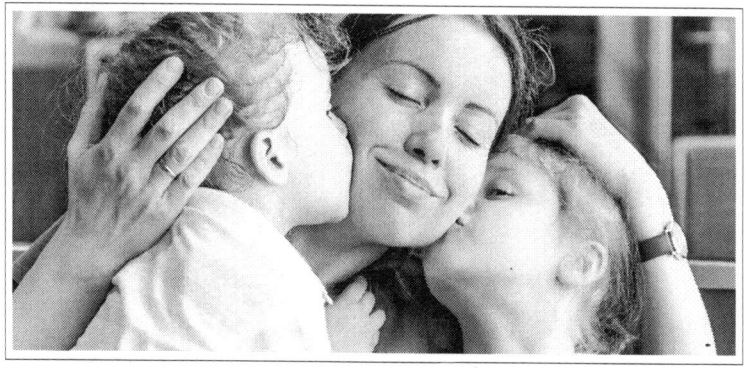

Indulge in health and happiness.

Poor excuses for poor eating habits

excuse	rebuttal
I don't have time.	You have this book and many others to help save time. Like any new thing, it takes more time at first but gets easier the more you do it.
I can't afford it.	You can find bargains for dry goods online or shop at farmers' markets or stores like Trader Joe's to save money. Grow your own food. Consider buying less and eating less, especially if you can stand to lose a few pounds! Eat for fuel but not for gluttony.
I'm on the road and often eat lunch on the run.	Keep a small cooler in your car for lunch and healthy snacks. Ask your favorite deli shop if they offer lettuce wraps with GF deli meat.
No way! I can't give up gluten [or insert your food culprit]!	Remember your body is for keeps, not for rent, as Julia Turshen reminds us in *It's All Good*, which she wrote with Gwyneth Paltrow. So, think twice before complaining about how you feel, if you haven't tried changing your diet — the one thing you have so much control over and that's so directly related.
The rest of my family won't get on board.	Maybe not right away. But if you do it and they see you feeling better, they will think twice about it and hopefully begin taking baby steps.

Let's consider these excuses as burps in your first attempt to digest this matter. Chew on it a little more until you're ready to take a bigger bite into eating healthier.

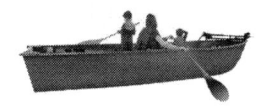

12. now for dessert — sweet stories of success

Finally, journey through these testimonials from just my small circle of contacts who have experienced either noticeable results or astounding differences by changing their diets. May these healthier eaters inspire and encourage you to do the same.

Theresa

Female, age 52

I am BRCA positive and previvor. BRCA refers to gene mutations that increase the risk of breast and ovarian cancer. A previvor is a survivor of a predisposition to cancer, often through a genetic mutation or a family history, who has not had the cancer. I had a double mastectomy and total hysterectomy to help prevent getting breast or ovarian cancer.

I was struggling with fatigue, frequent respiratory infections, joint swelling and pain. I don't want to ever have to go through chemo or radiation, and having the BRCA diagnosis, I decided to control what I can — which is what I put into my body.

Within a week of being off gluten, my joint swelling and pain was noticeably better. The fatigue I have complained about for decades is gone. I notice when I go off my diet, it's just not worth it. It's easier for me to be good all the time than to try to take days off the diet and then get back on it. The bad food is really just not worth it, taste or symptom wise.

As a busy, single mom, working 2 jobs, it has been challenging. My family still gives me grief about my food being "healthy," but they've gotten used to it and expect it now.

I am the oldest of my generation who is BRCA positive and the only one who has not had a diagnosis of cancer. I attribute that to my diet and lifestyle changes I started over 20 years ago. I continue to eat healthier today, although I do drink wine, which is my weakness.

I eat very healthy at home where I have 100% control over my diet. I cook most of the time from scratch. I eat fresh fruits, veggies, healthy oils and clean meat — organic, grass-fed or free-range and without antibiotics or hormones. I avoid gluten, processed foods and sweetened drinks. Basically, I eat what rots and eat it before it does.

I found it's actually cheaper and usually easier to throw something simple together at home. I use the crockpot to make meals ahead of time, usually over the weekend. I get fresh produce delivered at work weekly and order clean meat online. This way, I have more time to cook, don't go into grocery stores very often and don't feel as tempted to bring bad stuff home.

Melissa

Female, age 43

I was dealing with several symptoms, including chronic sinus infections, joint pain and fatigue, heightened food sensitivities that resulted in hives, itching, stomach aches, nausea, brain fog and increased susceptibility to infections and colds. I was also diagnosed with early onset of cataracts due to the use of steroidal nasal sprays to combat my chronic sinus infections, according to ophthalmologists.

The use of antibiotics and antihistamines from an infant until age 35 has not helped my situation, and I refuse to take them any longer unless it's an emergency, as they only agitate and intensify issues with my digestion and create a vicious cycle of infections.

I felt better when I reduced grain and dairy in the past but continued to experience many uncomfortable symptoms. Trying to determine the cause for these symptoms was frustrating, since traditional lab tests for health conditions, including gluten intolerance, came back normal. Eventually, with the help of a holistic healthcare professional, I located a company that conducted a more sensitive type of lab test. The test results indicated gluten intolerance.

With this new information, I knew that I needed to remove gluten and wheat products from my diet. During my original change in diet, which included complete removal of gluten, wheat, caffeine, dairy and most sugars, it took just about a month to have clearer sinuses, dramatically increased energy, reduced stomach issues and less joint pain. Granted, I did endure temporary withdrawal symptoms, including fatigue, agitation, headaches and anxiety when removing some of these foods. These lasted from a few days to a couple of weeks.

Then, after approximately six months on that diet, I decided to slowly begin eating some of the restricted foods and gradually experienced the same health issues but on an even greater level. So, I've reverted to a diet closer to the original one, without gluten or wheat, and have seen improvement in my health again.

I continue to use raw sugar rather than refined sugar, if needed, and completely avoid artificial sweeteners. I have removed nightshades, which give me heartburn and acid reflux. I've reduced intake of all grains, caffeine and dairy products, especially those with high lactose content. And I continue to eat more fresh, organic and locally grown foods.

Fortunately, it's pretty simple to eat at home but a bit more difficult to eat at restaurants, friends' homes or social gatherings. I've learned to ask lots of questions as well as get over the embarrassment of feeling like a pain!

So, I'm still eating a limited diet, because it is critical to my long-term health. I have talked with many individuals who have had similar health concerns that resulted in kidney and pancreatic damage or other long-term health issues, because they didn't realize that changing their diets could help. There are so many good foods that I can still eat, so I don't miss the others as much now. And the foods that I'm sensitive to are not worth eating if they compromise my overall health.

Ron

Male, age 61

Around 25 years ago, I would get large hives on my body that would last 10 days. I went to 3 different dermatologists, who suggested hydrocortisone and dapsone, which would require a test each year to monitor potential damage to my liver.

Finally, about 7 years ago, my primary care doctor decided to test me for celiac disease, and the test came back positive. It took 6 or 7 months of being gluten free, but the hives did go away.

If I eat gluten by mistake, I may get a hive, even up to as long as a month after exposure to it, and it can still last 5 or 6 days.

Now instead of gluten, I eat more vegetables, potatoes and some gluten-free products.

Rebecca

Female, age 41

I suffered from Hashimoto's hypothyroidism, dealing with symptoms of brain fog, fatigue and slow metabolism. I adopted a gluten-free diet and in about a month, my lab work came back normal after initially having high anti-thyroid antibodies. My symptoms, particularly the brain fog, also improved.

After 3 years of eating gluten free, I did end up needing to start a low dose thyroid medicine. But I still eat gluten free because I don't want to stress my thyroid. Eating gluten free helps me avoid eating junk and forces me to be more mindful of what I eat.

Niki

Female, age 34

I felt sick often, and my son had hyperactivity and seizures. I took out all grains, gluten, legumes, soy and processed foods. Then I added lots of organic vegetables, fruits, grass-fed beef, free-range chicken and eggs, wild-caught fish, raw dairy, bone broth, organ meats and fermented foods.

Very quickly I saw results. My family is rarely sick anymore. We have more energy and glowing skin. My son's seizures went away without medicines, and he is so much calmer — almost like a new kid!

My biggest challenges in eating healthier were relearning how to cook, getting the kids on board and spending more money on foods. However, we have nearly no costs for over-the-counters or doctor visits.

We're definitely still eating this way and still learning and getting better about making healthy choices at events and parties instead of just in our home.

Jamie

Male, age 42

My wife has tried several diets for her allergies, and I agreed to go gluten free with her for 3 weeks to see if it made any difference in how I felt. Plus, I figured I could stand to lose a few pounds.

Giving up beer was the most difficult part for me. I drank an occasional gluten-free beer or vodka cocktail. For lunch, I ate more salads. I felt hungrier throughout the day, too.

I didn't notice much change in how I felt. However, I did lose 12 pounds in 3 weeks. I will do it again just to give my body a break and to force myself to eat healthier again.

Bev

Female, age 56

I had been diagnosed with polymyositis, which is chronic muscle inflammation accompanied by muscle weakness. I also had arthritis and high cholesterol while being overweight. I struggled with inflammation, shortness of breath, depression, overall weakness, swelling and fatigue.

I removed soda and all whites — breads, pastas, sugar, flour, dairy, meats. I added water intake and 30 minutes of moderate exercise most days. This began as an effort in my church to do a variation of the "Daniel fast." I noticed less inflammation and pain within just 3 days. It's that quick!

I also lost about 20 pounds in that 23-day period.

I've done other diets over the years, too, at times losing as many as 55 pounds and keeping them off for almost 2 years. But my challenge is maintaining the diets. The muscle disease makes it difficult to exercise, and the steroids I take periodically for it make it difficult to keep weight off and swelling down. I wear orthopedics because I have flat feet and suffer from plantar fasciitis. I also have hip, back and disc problems. Most of my symptoms lessen or disappear after I start eating right and losing weight. But a busy schedule and high-stress account management job steer me into drive-throughs too often.

Each year, I do the fast for 23 days and say I'm going to continue it, while adding chicken and fish. But my busy lifestyle puts me off track, typically a few weeks into that effort. I know I want to eat healthier but need to find ways to make it easier.

Laurie

Female, age 59

I was suffering from acid reflux, irritable bowel syndrome (IBS) and hiatal hernia while taking 5 medicines each day just to eat. I felt awful a good part of my day with burning, bloating and diarrhea, and doctors said I would be on the meds for life.

My mother died from stomach cancer when she was 39 and I was 11. When I became pregnant with my own daughter at 39, I knew that I had to change course and that the human body could heal on its own. I knew the best gift I could give my daughter was to stay alive.

The first day I figured this out, I gave up coffee, and the next day my stomach wasn't on fire, burning and bloated. So, I thought, "Wow, if just this one thing could make me feel that much better, what if I kept going?" So, I gave up all fried foods, then red meat, soda, sweets and so on. I ate vegetarian for 7 years and have eaten vegan for the past 4 years.

Because I had instant results and continued to feel so much better month-by-month and year-by-year, eating healthier didn't seem so challenging. I love it and feel great. I got off all prescription and over-the-counter medicines within months and have stayed off of them for over a decade, now symptom free after 20 years. My endoscopies/colonoscopies show I'm clear of inflammation, which my doctors thought they'd never see.

I have lots of energy, don't get colds or flus and never feel sick. I'm exercising most days of the week, power walking and lifting weights, healthier at 60 than I was in my 20s. I also left corporate America after a 25-year career to help people reach a healthy weight as a Certified Health Coach and Licensed HeartMath® Stress Reduction Coach to learn about the amazing HeartMath technology, which monitors your physical and emotional health, as well as the HeartMath stress reduction tools, which help you improve them.

I live the habits of health rather than the habits of disease. Let food be thy medicine and medicine be thy food, along with stress reduction tools! The body will heal on its own when given healthy inputs.

It's been a wonderful journey.

Please share your stories, ideas and encouragement at facebook.com/digestedbook and leave your review at digestedbook.com.

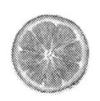

just one more bite

Indeed. It has been a wonderful journey. Even though I'm still venturing for better health, I've experienced the glory of taking many winding, scenic side roads to learn how to feed my body more naturally. Not just natural in the sense of organic, but with respect to how foods interact with my body at this exact time in my life and as it continues to change.

Throughout my life, I've tried to control many things to improve my health — allergies, stress, others' behaviors, my own reactions, emotions, environment. But now I've realized that this is like bandaging my symptoms instead of truly mending my wound. Instead, by eating healthier, I can begin to heal my damaged body while making it more resilient to all of those symptomatic elements that are outside my control.

I've also learned that contrary to my instincts and habits, I need to give control of my worries, stress and destination over to God. As I grow in my renewed faith, I anticipate even greater results from eating healthier and treating my body like a temple — as He intends for us to do.

If you digest only one tidbit from this book, let it be this — you have the power and means to help improve your health simply by choosing to eat healthier.

To what extreme you take that is up to you. The magnitude of improvement you feel remains to be seen. The number of people influenced by your decision could be exponential. And you get to explore and enjoy a new perspective of foods all along the way.

Here's to eating healthier and to sunnier days ahead.

— *Natalie Gensits*

Notes — reasons I choose to eat healthier

Symptoms I have and things I want to research more

New foods or kitchen tools to try

Works cited

Chapter 3

Ungar, Laura. "Pre-diabetes, diabetes rates fuel national health crisis." *Usatoday.com*. September 15, 2014. http://www.usatoday.com/story/news/nation/2014/09/14/prediabetesrising-diabetes-threatening-usa/15134489/.

Kharrazian, Datis, DHSc, DC, MS. *Why Do I Still Have Thyroid Symptoms? When My Lab Tests are Normal.* Carlsbad, California: Elephant Press, 2010. 119.

Bond, Geoff. *Natural Eating, Nutritional Anthropology: Eating in Harmony with our Genetic Programming.* Torrance, California: Griffin Publishing Group, 2000. 112.

Fragoso, Sarah. *Everyday Paleo.* Las Vegas, Nevada: Victory Belt Publishing, 2011. 26.

"Human Digestive System." *Enchantedlearning.com*. July 8, 2015. http://www.enchantedlearning.com/subjects/anatomy/digestive/.

Zimmermann, Kim Ann. "Digestive System: Facts, Function & Diseases." *LiveScience.com*. April 22, 2015. http://www.livescience.com/22367-digestive-system.html.

Chapter 4

"GMO Defined." *Gmo-awareness.com*. July 8, 2015. http://gmo-awareness.com/all-about-gmos/gmo-defined/.

Merriam-Webster. *Merriam-webster.com*. July 8, 2015. http://www.merriamwebster.com/dictionary/whole%20foods.

"Organic Labeling." *Usda.gov*. December 5, 2012. http://www.ams.usda.gov/AMSv1.0/ams.fetchTemplateData.do?template=TemplateA&navID=OrgLabelingLinkNOPOrganicLabeling&rightNav1=OrgLabelingLinkNOPOrganicLabeling&topNav=&leftNav=NationalOrganicProgram&page=NOPOrganicLabeling&resultType=&acct=nopgeninfo.

"The 'Non-GMO Project Verified' Seal." *Nongmoproject.org*. July 8, 2015. http://www.nongmoproject.org/learn-more/understanding-our-seal/.

"National Organic Program." *Ams.usda.gov*. Updated May 29, 2015. http://www.ams.usda.gov/AMSv1.0/ams.fetchTemplateData.do?template=TemplateC&leftNav=NationalOrganicProgram&page=NOP-Consumers&description=Consumers.

"What is the meaning of 'natural' on the label of food?" *Fda.gov.* April 29, 2015. http://www.fda.gov/aboutfda/transparency/basics/ucm214868.htm.

"National Organic Program." *Ams.usda.gov.* Updated May 29, 2015. http://www.ams.usda.gov/AMSv1.0/ams.fetchTemplateData.do?template=TemplateC&leftNav=NationalOrganicProgram&page=NOP-Consumers&description=Consumers.

"Identifying Whole Grain Products." *Wholegrainscouncil.org.* July 9, 2015. http://wholegrainscouncil.org/whole-grains-101/identifying-whole-grain-products.

Bond, Geoff. *Natural Eating, Nutritional Anthropology: Eating in Harmony with our Genetic Programming.* Torrance, California: Griffin Publishing Group, 2000. 116-118.

"Conjugated Linoleic Acid". *Webmd.com.* July 8, 2015. http://www.webmd.com/vitamins-supplements/ingredientmono-826-conjugated%20linoleic%20acid.aspx?activeingredientid=826&activeingredientname=conjugated%20linoleic%20acid.

Nelson, Jennifer K., R.D., L.D. "What is high-fructose corn syrup? What are the health concerns?" *Mayoclinic.org.* September 27, 2012. http://www.mayoclinic.org/healthyliving/nutrition-and-healthy-eating/expert-answers/high-fructose-corn-syrup/faq-20058201.

Chapter 5

"Sodium in Your Diet: Using the Nutrition Facts Label to Reduce Your Intake." *Fda.gov.* Last updated May 7, 2015. http://www.fda.gov/Food/ResourcesForYou/Consumers/ucm315393.htm.

Kresser, Chris. "Shaking Up The Salt Myth: Healthy Salt Recommendations." *Chriskresser.com.* May 4, 2012. http://chriskresser.com/shaking-up-the-salt-myth-healthy-salt-recommendations/.

Nelson, Jennifer K., R.D., L.D. "What is high-fructose corn syrup? What are the health concerns?" *Mayoclinic.org.* September 27, 2012. http://www.mayoclinic.org/healthyliving/nutrition-and-healthy-eating/expert-answers/high-fructose-corn-syrup/faq-20058201.

Mercola, Joseph, D.O. "Sugar Substitutes – What's Safe and What's Not." *Articles.mercola.com.* October 7, 2013. http://articles.mercola.com/sites/articles/archive/2013/10/07/sugar-substitutes.aspx.

Walton, Allison G. "How Much Sugar Are Americans Eating? [Infographic]." *Forbes.com*. August 30, 2012. http://www.forbes.com/sites/alicegwalton/2012/08/30/how-much-sugar-are-americans-eating-infographic/.

Nordqvist, Joseph. "How much sugar is in your food?" *Medicalnewstoday.com*. June 16, 2014. http://www.medicalnewstoday.com/articles/262978.php.

Chapter 6

Lee, Stephanie L., MD, PhD. "Hashimoto Thyroiditis." *Medscape.com*. June 3, 2014. http://emedicine.medscape.com/article/120937-overview.

"Array 4 – Gluten-Associated Cross-Reactive Foods and Foods Sensitivity." *Cyrexlabs.com*. 2015. http://www.cyrexlabs.com/CyrexTestsArrays/tabid/136/Default.aspx.

Myers, Amy, MD. "Are You Not Healing Because Your Body Thinks Coffee, Chocolate & Cheese Are Gluten?" *Mindbodygreen.com*. February 28, 2013. http://www.mindbodygreen.com/0-7875/are-you-not-healing-because-your-body-thinks-coffee-chocolate-cheese-are-glute.html.

Ballantyne, Sarah, PhD. "Gluten Cross-Reactivity UPDATE: How your body can still think you're eating gluten even after giving it up." *Thepaleomom.com*. March 13, 2013. http://www.thepaleomom.com/2013/03/gluten-cross-reactivity-update-how-your-body-can-still-think-youre-eating-gluten-even-after-giving-it-up.html.

Paltrow, Gwyneth and Julia Turshen. *It's All Good*. New York, New York: Grand Central Life & Style, Hachette Book Group, 2013. 14.

Dengate, Sue. "Food Intolerance Network Factsheet – Amines". *Food Intolerance Network*. August 2006. http://fedup.com.au/factsheets/additive-and-natural-chemical-factsheets/amines.

Anne, Melodie. "Symptoms of Coffee Allergies." *Livestrong.com*. April 15, 2015. http://www.livestrong.com/article/45331-symptoms-coffee-allergies/.

Daniluk, Julie, R.H.N. *Meals That Heal Inflammation*. Carlsbad, California: Hay House, Inc., 2011. 46.

Zelman, Kathleen M., MPH, RD, LD. "Food Allergies and Food Intolerance." *Webmd.com*. February 11, 2014. http://www.webmd.com/allergies/guide/food-allergyintolerances?.

Marks, Diane. "Allergies to Nightshade Vegetables." *Livestrong.com*. Feb 18, 2015. http://www.livestrong.com/article/320713-allergies-to-nightshade-vegetables/.

"Types of Food Allergy – Peanut Allergy". *Acaai.org*. July 8, 2015. http://acaai.org/allergies/types/food-allergies/types-food-allergy/peanut-allergy.

"Pork Allergy." *Activeonehealth.com*. July 8, 2015. http://www.activeonehealth.com/viewarticle.php?artid=5.

"Types of Food Allergy – Soy Allergy." *Acaai.org*. July 8, 2015. http://acaai.org/allergies/types/food-allergies/types-food-allergy/soy-allergy.

Seidu, Luqman, MD. "Asthma and Sulfite Allergies." *Webmd.com*. January 18, 2015. http://www.webmd.com/asthma/asthma-and-sulfites-allergies.

"Types of Food Allergy – Wheat Allergy." *Acaai.org*. July 8, 2015. http://acaai.org/allergies/types/food-allergies/types-food-allergy/wheat-gluten-allergy.

Daniluk, Julie, R.H.N. *Meals That Heal Inflammation*. Carlsbad, California: Hay House, Inc., 2011. 60.

"Simple Substitutions." *Simply Gluten Free Magazine*, July-August 2014. 64.

Daniluk, Julie, R.H.N. *Meals That Heal Inflammation*. Carlsbad, California: Hay House, Inc., 2011. 209-211.

Koeller Kim and Robert La France. *Let's Eat Out with Celiac/Coeliac & Food Allergies*. Chicago, Illinois: Gluten Free Passport, 2011.

Kresser, Chris. "How too much omega-6 and not enough omega-3 is making us sick." *Chriskresser.com*. May 8, 2010. http://chriskresser.com/how-too-much-omega-6-and-not-enough-omega-3-is-making-us-sick/.

Davidson, Emily. *101 Natural Healthy Eating Tips*. Boston, Massachusetts: LifeTips.com, Inc., 2008. 77.

Daniluk, Julie, R.H.N. *Meals That Heal Inflammation*. Carlsbad, California: Hay House, Inc., 2011. 78.

Chapter 7

Fragoso, Sarah. *Everyday Paleo*. Las Vegas, Nevada: Victory Belt Publishing, 2011. 15.

Chapter 10

Bond, Geoff. *Natural Eating, Nutritional Anthropology: Eating in Harmony with our Genetic Programming*. Torrance, California: Griffin Publishing Group, 2000. 100, 103.

"Heart-Healthy Cooking: Oils 101." *Health Hub from Cleveland Clinic*. October 1, 2014. http://health.clevelandclinic.org/2014/10/heart-healthy-cooking-oils-101/.

Urban, Shilo. "How to Cook with Oils: The Manifesto." *Organicauthority.com*. September 20, 2010. http://www.organicauthority.com/eco-chic-table/guide-to-cooking-with-oils.html.

"To Nuke or Not to Nuke? Should You Microwave Your Food?" *The Oz Blog*. April 15, 2013. http://blog.doctoroz.com/oz-experts/to-nuke-or-not-to-nuke-should-you-microwave-your-food.

Brown, Carolyn, MS, RD. "Open Your Mind (and Your Mouth) to New Foods." *Webmd.com*. September 23, 2013. http://blogs.webmd.com/food-and-nutrition/2013/09/open-your-mind-and-your-mouth-to-new-foods.html.

Index

100% whole grain, 22, 69
ADD (attention deficit disorder), 9, 23
additives, 3, 6, 48
ADHD (attention deficit hyperactivity disorder), 2, 23, 47
alkaloid, 30, 48
almond, 55, 62, 73
amines, 47-48
antibiotics, 2, 11, 31, 44
aspartame, 35, 36, 48
autoimmune, 8, 24, 32, 41, 59
bisphenol A (BPA), 33, 79, 82
bread, 12, 22-23, 31, 53-54
breakfast, 12, 30, 54, 64, 82
caffeine, 9, 33, 58, 90
cage-free, 21
calcium, 9, 56
canned (foods), 27, 36, 72, 80
casein, 24-25, 43, 50, 63
cayenne, 48, 59
celiac disease, 12, 43, 55, 90
certified organic, 18-19, 31, 71
chocolate, 36, 43, 52
cinnamon, 59
coconut water, 56, 73
coffee, 37, 43, 47, 58, 93
constipation, 32, 35, 41, 47, 56
cookware, 79
cross-reactors, 42-43
culprit, 12, 40, 43, 46, 55
digestion, 10
dinner, 2, 54, 65, 75
dyes, 38, 48
ear infection, 2, 68-69
electrolytes, 11, 33, 56
elimination (diet), 43
enzymes, 10, 24-27, 40, 48
estrogen-mimicking, 79

evaporated cane juice, 26
fermented foods, 32, 48, 91
fiber, 24, 26, 56
flora, 11-12, 32, 57
food allergy, 39-40, 46
free-range, 21, 31, 72, 88, 91
fructose, see also sugar, 27, 34, 36
fruits, 12, 27, 30, 36, 65, 68, 71, 77
garlic, 51, 59
genetic modification, 17
gluten, 2, 12, 23, 42-43, 47, 50, 53-55, 64
gluten-free, 6, 53-55, 65, 72-73, 91
GMOs (genetically modified organisms), 15, 17, 23, 30, 53
grains, 2, 21-24, 30, 53-54, 61, 63, 69
grass-fed, 21, 31, 62, 88
Hashimoto's disease, 41-42
high fructose corn syrup (HFCS), 27, 36
hyperactivity, 2, 9, 15, 38, 47
hypothyroidism, 8, 41-42, 91
inflammation, 5, 8, 11, 30, 32, 43, 46-48, 59
intolerance, 12, 23, 25, 38-41, 43, 49, 89
iodine, 56
iron, 56, 59
irritable bowel syndrome (IBS), 32, 47, 93
juice concentrate, 22, 71
kohlrabi, 29, 52, 54, 77
labels, 17, 31, 53, 71, 74
lactose, 25, 63
leaky gut syndrome, 32, 41, 44
lectin, 48
legume, 21, 52, 61, 63, 72
lunch, 55, 65
magnesium, 26, 56, 73
meal preparation, 75

microwave, 33, 82
milk, 2, 24-26, 31, 43, 50, 57, 68
mucous membranes, 11-12, 44, 46
multi-grain, 22
mushroom, 59, 71
natural, 20, 22
nightshades, 8, 30, 47, 48, 90
nitrates, 31
Non-GMO Project verified, 19, 20, 23
nutrients, 8-12, 56-57, 82
nuts, 47, 48, 51, 56, 62, 69, 72
oil, 17, 31, 61-63, 72, 74, 80-81
omega-3, 55, 57
omega-6, 55, 73, 81
organic, 18-20, 30-31, 71-73
papaya, 59
pasture-raised, 21, 31, 62
plastic, 15, 33, 79
poop, 8, 11, 45
potassium, 9, 48, 57, 73, 78
potato, 30, 43, 47, 48, 52, 62-63, 78
probiotics, 26, 31-32, 57, 68
protein, 10, 26, 31, 48, 78
salt, see also sodium, 34, 63
sensitivity, 40, 48
sesame, 43, 56, 59, 73
shopping list, 72-73
snack, 37-38, 52, 54, 65
sodium, see also salt, 34, 48, 57, 63
soy, 17, 26-27, 31, 43, 47, 51, 56, 63
spices, 59, 63
starch, 13, 52, 54, 77-78
sugar, 2, 27, 34-37, 52
sugar substitutes, 8, 35-36
sulfites, 47, 48
sweet potato, 30, 50, 59, 62, 68
tartrazine, see also yellow 5, 38, 48
thyroid, 8, 23, 41-42
toxicity, 39-40
turmeric, 59

tyramine, 48
unbleached flour, 23
USDA organic, 18-20
vegetables, 30, 62, 68, 71, 77
villi, 12
vinegar, 32, 51, 80
vitamin D, 57
washing foods, 80
water, 15, 32-33, 68, 79
weight-loss, 8
whole food, 18
whole grain, 17, 22-24, 69
withdrawal symptoms, 5, 55, 89
yellow 5, see also tartrazine, 14, 38, 47-49
yerba mate, 58

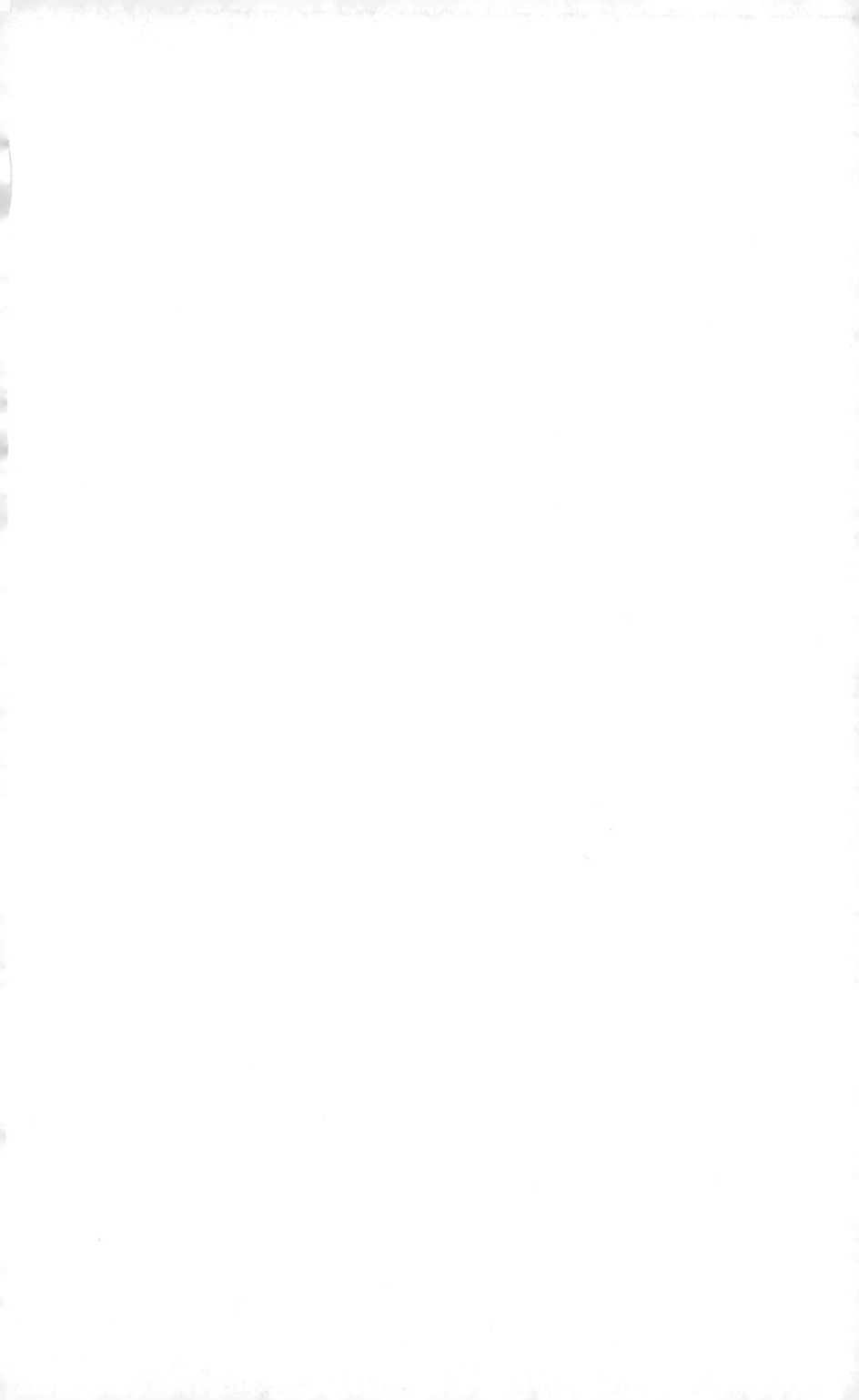

Made in the USA
San Bernardino, CA
29 February 2016